Overpower Pain

OVERPOWER PAIN

*The Strength-Training Program that
Stops Pain Without Drugs or Surgery*

Mitchell T. Yass, PT

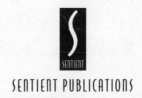

SENTIENT PUBLICATIONS

First Sentient Publications edition 2008
Copyright © 2008 by Mitchell T. Yass

A paperback original

Cover design by Andrew Brozyna
Book design by Timm Bryson
Photographs by Rosanna Wolff

Library of Congress Cataloging-in-Publication Data

Yass, Mitchell T, 1961-
  Overpower pain : the strength-training program that stops pain without
drugs or surgery / by Mitchell T. Yass.
    p. cm.
 ISBN 978-1-59181-075-9
 1. Weight training–Therapeutic use. I. Title.

RM725.Y37 2008
615.5'3–dc22

                            2007051837

Printed in the United States of America

10 9 8 7 6 5 4 3 2 1

SENTIENT PUBLICATIONS
A Limited Liability Company
1113 Spruce Street
Boulder, CO 80302
www.sentientpublications.com

To my wife Lioa. I want to thank her for standing by me in good times and bad. She has been both a rock to cling to and a stream of tranquility to soothe me. She has been the best thing to ever come into my life. She has completed my soul by giving me my beautiful daughter, Natalya Rose. I dedicate this book to them.

Contents

Preface

It is important for you to understand the context from which this book arose, how it should be used, and under what conditions it should be used. It is a synopsis of the diagnostic rules I use to differentiate whether a patient's symptoms are the result of muscle weakness or if they are caused by structural problems such as a herniated disc or arthritis. If the cause is muscular weakness, the only way to resolve this cause is through strength training. This book provides specific exercises to resolve pain at each joint of the body including the neck and lower back.

If the pain is structural, medical intervention is needed. No form of exercise will resolve symptoms caused by *structural deficits*. I believe that there are cases where the cause is structural and medical intervention is necessary. I have had years of experience treating patients who were improperly diagnosed with structural causes for their pain. This led to treatment protocols incorporating medication and pain management, and in many cases, surgery was deemed necessary. I diagnosed the cause as muscular using the techniques described in this book, and the patients were placed on treatment plans incorporating aggressive strength training. The patients' symptoms were resolved and all forms of treatment ended.

A pattern has developed where muscular causes are not recognized until patients come to me for treatment. It is imperative that

information regarding the diagnosis of muscular symptoms be provided to the general public. This book can be used as a reference
for the diagnosis of muscular symptoms, or it can be used to facilitate dialogue between patient and physician resulting in more
effective treatment.

We must distinguish the type of pain discussed here from other
types of pain. The pain described in this book pertains to injuries where some form of trauma caused inflammation, resulting in
muscle, tendon, or joint pain. Trauma does not necessarily imply
one specific incident such as a fall or sudden injury. Trauma refers
to injuries that occur over sustained periods of time, such as those
caused by repetitive activity like hammering, or basic activities like
walking or standing for sustained periods when the individual was
not conditioned for them. The majority of my patients are unable to
identify a specific cause of their pain. This shows that the cause of
pain associated with traumatic forces does not have to be extreme
to lead to a breakdown of tissues. This type of pain is different
from systemic causes of pain resulting from diseases such as can-
cer, kidney and gallstones, or other visceral dysfunctions. The book
does not attempt to differentiate between these two main causes
of pain. If you believe that the origin of your pain is systemic, you
should certainly seek medical care. But if the symptoms are similar
to those described in the book, identifying the cause of pain as
muscular, then you should try the exercises to resolve the pain.

You should get approval from your family physician before beginning any exercise program to make sure that there are no con-
traindications prohibiting exercise.

Once you have this approval, you should use the book to determine which exercises to perform to achieve your goals, whether it
is the resolution of pain at a certain joint or just for general conditioning purposes. Do not try to use the weights being displayed in
the start and finish photos when starting to use the exercises. The
photos are for reference to show proper form. To determine the

proper weight to use when performing the exercises, please follow the instructions in the book.

Strength training should not feel awkward. The movements should be fairly simple and you should be stable to prevent injury. If the exercises are followed properly and the correct weight is used to perform them, you should achieve strength safely and effectively, correcting the appropriate weakness or muscle imbalance and ultimately resolving the pain.

I was always exceptionally thin—the proverbial ninety-nine-pound weakling—until I was well into my twenties. From nineteen until twenty-six, I tried lifting weights to get bigger and to improve my poor self-esteem. I'd take out the weights, and, for three to six months, I'd use them, but nothing would happen. I would work out only at home, because I was so self-conscious about how thin I was.

Finally, when I was twenty-six, I started to see improvement, and, by the time I was thirty, I'd put on forty pounds of muscle. I've continued to lift for the past twenty years and have put on ten additional pounds of muscle over the years. But the benefits I've received from **weight training** (boldfaced, italicized words can be found in the glossary) have been more than just physical. Over time, my self-esteem has improved dramatically as well. My belief that I can overcome obstacles with hard work and dedication stems from my experience with weight lifting. I now have a level of confidence that inspires people around me to do their best. When I speak about weight training, I have the kind of credibility that comes from life experience.

The confidence I gained from my personal awakening through **weight lifting** has carried over to my career. In my **physical therapy** practice, I deal with a lot of sports-related injuries and also offer personal training. Because of this, I feel that my appearance is important. The best way to teach is by example. When I work with people one-on-one, my appearance reinforces my instruction. I've worked successfully with one or two professional athletes, and high school and college athletes also respond well to me. They value what I tell them, because my appearance is proof that it works.

Weight training has also improved my concentration level. When I am lifting extremely heavy weights, concentration becomes very important to perform the exercise correctly. Even the slightest deviation can result in using muscles unprepared for such resistance, and serious injury can result.

Yet, I've never had an injury. I've been able to extend this improved level of concentration to other areas of my life, such as my physical therapy practice. I often work with six or seven patients simultaneously. These can include neurological, orthopedic, post-surgical, and accident cases. It requires a high level of concentration and discipline to know exactly what's going on with each patient when I'm working with so many at once, yet I now find it very easy to focus on information such as what exercises or weights the patients are using or to what extent they have progressed.

As for discipline, I've weight trained continually for more than twenty years, and I have no intention of stopping. In fact, I'm more excited about weight lifting now than I've ever been. The discipline I've gained extends to other parts of my life, and it can for you as well. Weight training can teach you to stay with something for the long haul, whether it's maintaining a relationship or sticking with a job and growing in the position. Weight training proves that hard work pays off and leads to success. It's a tough lesson, but the rewards are enormous. For me, going from 160 pounds when I was in my twenties to my current weight of 210 wasn't simply about gaining the weight; it was about wanting to change something about myself and succeeding. Even though I was working against my naturally thin body type, my will, determination, and fortitude allowed me to achieve great success.

Of course, publishing this book tops that. I wrote the book primarily because I wanted to share the experiences of the patients I've worked with. I wanted to explain how these exercises both corrected their injuries and improved their quality of life by helping them to feel better. My intention is not just to help my patients heal, but to help them live without Monday morning pain. I use my experiences with weight training to motivate patients, explaining how, through hard work, I overcame my predisposition to be thin. My patients overcome their injuries the same way. Through weight training, they correct muscle strength imbalances, which, the majority of the time, are the source of pain. Once the patients become stronger, they have a better chance of limiting injuries.

Even today, with all the interest in staying in shape, many people believe weight training is just for the young—something people do just to look better. There's so much more to it than that. If I can help you understand that even the most basic weight-training program can help you feel better, then my purpose for writing this book will be fulfilled.

I hope my experience as a *physical therapist* will encourage you to take my vision of weight training more seriously than if I were a celebrity or well-known bodybuilder relying on simply trial and error. My knowledge of injury prevention and proper technique can help you feel confident that what I'm telling you is correct, so you'll be more apt to try it. Because I incorporate my training experience and my educational and professional backgrounds, this book describes one of the safest weight-training programs available.

The benefits you will receive are many. Strengthening your muscles builds bone mass, which prevents *osteoporosis*. What's more, the greater your muscle mass, the more efficient your body will be at burning fat. And no matter what activities you participate in, whether you're a weekend gardener or a triathlete, building muscle balance prevents injury. If you've always wanted to start a weight-training program but lacked quality information to get you started, this book is the answer. The information comes from both scientific sources and through feedback from people similar to you who have experienced the value of exercise at my facility. They've used it not only to heal injuries, but also as a means of feeling better in general. The message is clear: everybody should be lifting weights. When will you begin?

1

WEIGHT LIFTING ISN'T JUST FOR BODYBUILDERS

As a physical therapist, I find that patients do much better when they understand what goes on while they exercise. Weight training, regardless of the injury, is necessary to complete a patient's rehabilitation, even if the injury or condition required surgical intervention. At some point after an injury or surgery, the affected body part is immobilized and the surrounding musculature becomes weak. Some mobility is lost. Whether a patient receives ice, *electrical stimulation*, or some other form of treatment (*massage*, *ultrasound*, etc.), he must stretch and strengthen to restore normal functioning to the affected area. Our natural tendency is to stop using an injured body part to avoid pain. As a result, swelling may occur due to decreased muscular *contractile force*, which is the main factor in limiting fluid buildup. Surrounding muscles weaken, and pain develops. I work with patients of all ages, from children as young as six to people in their nineties, and no matter what age the patients are, I use *progressive resistance weight training* to correct their deficits. The more information patients have regarding the purpose of strength training, which muscles they are working and how, the more motivated and successful they are, and the more likely they are to achieve recovery.

Exercise not only helps my patients to recover from their injuries, but it also benefits them long after they're discharged. For example, if you stop lifting, the muscles could weaken and the injury could recur. Higher levels of physical fitness can also enhance your quality of life by improving your *cardiovascular* and *immune systems*, according to recent studies (Judy Foreman, *Globe* staff, 1996; Kevin R. Vincent MD, PhD; Heather K. Vincent PhD, 2006)[1].

When you exercise, your cardiovascular and *pulmonary systems* supply increased amounts of blood and oxygen to the working muscles and remove the byproduct of muscular contraction, *lactic acid*. Lactic acid alters the ph of the blood which can affect systemic function.

As you continue to exercise over a period of time, these systems become more efficient. Your body temperature also rises as a result of exercise, causing a release of white blood cells, which protect the body from invading bacteria and viruses. **Strength training** can also limit the typical aches and pains associated with weekend activities such as household chores, gardening, and athletic endeavors. Physical inactivity during the course of the week contributes to the nagging injuries of the "weekend warrior." These are often unnecessary, recurrent injuries.

The most interesting thing about correcting these injuries is the way people realize they're getting better. Instead of being aware of feeling stronger or being able to move a joint more freely, they notice they can now comb their hair, tie their shoes, or perform some other activity that previously had caused them pain. Even if you don't have specific injuries, proper weight training will allow you to breeze through daily chores without aches and pains and still have energy to enjoy more pleasurable activities.

Probably my most rewarding case of a person resolving an injury through strength training involved a twenty-six-year-old man with an extremely severe case of *sciatica.* The patient installs roofing for a living, which requires carrying hundred-pound rolls of tar paper on his shoulder up to a roof. He also uses a rope to hoist hundreds of cans of tar weighing close to one hundred pounds apiece. For two years, he'd been experiencing a burning sensation down the back of his leg, all the way down to his foot. He said it was as if someone were shooting his foot with a blowtorch, and it had progressed to the point where he was unable to work for six months.

His doctors diagnosed him with sciatica and prescribed painkillers. During the initial stages of his treatment, his mother told me he'd taken every conceivable painkiller, but the painkillers were no longer altering his pain level. She also told me that he would spend hours lying on the floor, because he could find no other position or place that was comfortable. If my suggested therapy of moist heat, massage, and weight lifting didn't help, doctors were considering surgery as a final means of eliminating his pain. During my evaluation, I concluded that his *sciatic nerve* had become inflamed as a result of an adjacent muscle that was thickening and compressing the nerve. This muscle thickened because many of the surrounding muscles were exceptionally weak, causing the muscle to overwork and break down.

The approach was simple: The patient performed an aggressive stretching and strengthening program to get his muscles working together, reducing the inflammation of the piriformis, taking pressure off of the sciatic nerve and eliminating his pain.

Within a couple of weeks, his symptoms began to subside. After a couple of months, he was able to return to work part time, and within ten months, he returned to full-time work. All his symptoms have now completely disappeared, and tasks at work have become much easier for him. He now challenges himself, pushing to see just how much more he can do with his newfound strength. Previously the movements he is now able to do could have resulted in injuries that would have kept him from work for a week. One of the nicest compliments I've received was being invited to his engagement party. He told me the engagement never would have been possible without my assistance.

Improvement of quality of life can occur at any age: the middle years, and even the sixties, seventies, and eighties. I had a seventy-four-year-old patient whose arm was so weak she had to hold it at the elbow with her left hand to put her car key into the ignition. At the end of six months of weight training and therapy, she was able to raise her arm through a full range of motion. Holding it up above her head, she was able to resist my applied force with a pretty good amount of force of her own. The fact that it took a seventy-four-year-old woman only six months to achieve this dramatically demonstrates that you can increase your strength at any age.

Another patient, an eighty-seven-year-old man, came in with a knee injury. He had severe emphysema and could walk only two or three steps without coughing up fluid. The strength training he performed to resolve his knee problem also greatly reduced the effects of his emphysema. Fluid buildup in his lungs was decreased, thereby improving his lung function. He could complete an entire exercise session without even a cough, and he was able to reduce by half the diuretic he was taking to limit fluid development. Nothing else was different—just exercise.

You wouldn't think it possible for people in their sixties, seventies, and eighties to become stronger, but the ability of muscle to become stronger doesn't seem to be affected by age. This is because of the innate contractile force of muscle that offsets the loss of elasticity of the connective tissue surrounding the muscle fibers. You can increase your strength at any age. And it's about more than just growing bigger muscles and looking better; it's about allowing you to go through your daily activities with a lower chance of injury. A study (Fiatarone, M.A.; Marks, E.C.; Ryan, N.D.; Merideth, C.N.;

Lipsitz, L.A.; and Evan, W.J., 1990)[2] published in 1990 in the *Journal of the American Medical Association* found that individuals over the age of ninety were able to increase muscle mass of the quadriceps (front thigh muscle) in an eight-week high-intensity resistance training program. Significantly, there was a correlation between the subjects' increased muscle mass and their ability to walk for longer periods of time. The authors of the study concluded that "high-resistance weight training leads to significant gains in muscle strength, size, and functional mobility among frail residents of nursing homes up to ninety-six years of age."

I have a sixty-two-year-old personal training client who, when she began, was the most out-of-condition person I've ever seen. The day she started, we gave her three exercises to perform with extremely light weights—military presses, hamstring curls, and triceps extensions. The muscles she worked were sore for four days, and she couldn't return to exercising until the following week. A few months after she started training, she was in a car accident and walked away from it without any pain. She was convinced that this was due to her improved physical condition. A year into her personal training, she now wears sleeveless shirts to show off her enhanced physique. At a recent family reunion, relatives were grabbing her arms to feel just how firm she'd become. Even at rest, her muscles are defined and separated. She's now outspoken about how weight training can change your body, your self-image, and the way you feel.

A big concern today is obesity. The National Institutes of Health now describes it as the number one killer among health problems with controllable causes, ahead of smoking. Obese individuals are at an increased risk for many diseases, including high blood pressure, coronary heart disease, *osteoarthritis*, type 2 *diabetes*, stroke, and some cancers.

Many people are obsessed with decreasing their caloric intake, believing the reduction will spark a sustained weight loss. Unfortunately, caloric reduction by itself does not work. The body eventually limits its energy expenditure to sustain such daily functions as breathing and digestion. So decreased caloric intake results in decreased caloric expenditure. Later, with an increase in caloric intake, the body won't burn the additional calories because caloric intake may be decreased once again. Now there is a surplus of calories, and your weight becomes greater than it was before you started your diet. This is why so many people who lose weight end up gaining it all back and more.

Weight training breaks the cycle by raising your resting **metabolic rate**—the amount of calories you burn to sustain life at rest. Studies prove that weight training serves this function better than aerobic activity (Campbell, W., M. Crim, V. Young and W. Evans, 1994; CE Broeder, KA Burrhus, LS Svanevik and JH Wilmore, 1992)[3]. Weight lifting is the only form of exercise that grows muscle—the key to increasing **metabolism**. Keeping more muscle tissue alive requires more energy, and the energy source for metabolism is fat. When you reduce the amount of calories you take in, your body requires additional calories to sustain the increased muscle mass. This combination of reduced caloric intake and increased calorie burn results in fat loss.

Weight training involves isolating individual muscle groups and strengthening them as efficiently as possible. With other forms of exercise, the idea is to use as many muscle groups as possible.

A rowing machine, for instance, incorporates the muscles of the buttocks (**glutes**), front and back thighs (**quadriceps** and **hamstrings,** respectively), upper and lower back, and arms and shoulders. If one muscle is weak, the others can compensate for it, and you can still perform the exercise. If you're playing a sport, you're not achieving complete and balanced strengthening of all muscle groups. When one muscle group works harder than others to perform an activity, an imbalance occurs. This causes stronger muscles to tighten, making them susceptible to overstretching.

Also, weaker muscles can be injured by their inability to create the force necessary to perform the activity. By adding a weight-training program to your sport or activity, you're balancing your strength and flexibility. This reduces the possibility of injury and improves your performance.

To be physically fit, you must have strength, flexibility, and stamina. Strength refers to the amount of force a muscle can exert through a certain range of motion. You gain strength through proper weight training. Flexibility comes from proper stretching techniques (see Chapter 6). And stamina, or endurance, relates to a muscle's ability to sustain a contraction over a period of time, determined by the cardiovascular system's ability to provide oxygen and energy to the contracting muscle. Endurance is increased through long-term, continuous activity such as running, cycling, or even walking.

Most people don't fully appreciate the value of walking. Because it increases your heart rate, it can help you to lose weight and improve your cardiovascular conditioning. It also benefits the discs of the spine. Because there's no direct blood supply to these *discs*, they get their nutrients through the *cerebrospinal fluid* within the spinal column. As you walk, each time your foot strikes the ground, the spine is compressed. As you release and move to the opposite foot, or while your foot is in the air, the spine springs back and the discs expand, just like sponges. Nutrients are absorbed into the discs. So, a very controlled, weight-bearing type of activity such as walking, where there's a compression and then a release of the spine, is a good opportunity for your discs to get nutrients and to maintain health. The same system of providing nutrients to the vertebral discs occurs with strength-training exercises.

Maximizing your strength, flexibility, and endurance allows your body to perform at its peak efficiency, whether you're performing household chores or running a marathon. If you're a woman and you're worried about getting too muscular, don't be. It's true that there's a linear relationship between improved strength and increased mass. If you improve your strength by 10 percent, you'll increase your **muscle mass** by 10 percent. You can't get stronger without creating more mass. But if you're concerned that you'll develop a man-size physique similar to those you see on female professional bodybuilding shows, you can relax. These women have incorporated testosterone into their regimens, to the point where their male hormone levels are substantially higher than even my own, enabling them to build unnatural amounts of mass. Testosterone is the key reason that men, on average, are more muscular than women. With only minimal amounts of testosterone present in the average woman, the average woman would find it almost impossible to put on enough muscle mass to cause concern. So getting too big should not be an issue when deciding to try weight training. In fact, it's more likely you'll lose inches. As a muscle gets stronger, it pulls in the surrounding tissue (John P. Porcari, Jennifer Miller, Kelly Cornwell, Carl Foster, Mark Gibson, Karen McLean, Tom Kernozek, 2005)[4]. As you get stronger, you actually lose inches in the area of the strengthened muscle.

Another misconception is that there's a single piece of equipment that can do everything for you and save you from spending a lot of time exercising. You can use it while watching TV, reading, or listening to the radio. First of all, there's no single piece of equipment that will let you isolate each individual muscle group the way a weight-training program can. Most of this equipment— whether it's a bicycle, a StairMaster, or a rowing machine—incorporates mass muscle groups. A single type of exercise equipment does not allow you to isolate muscle groups, so you'll never be able to maintain the balance required for a good level of fitness. Forget the notion that exercise can or should be fun. You should do it because it offers such a tremendous value to you.

2

BE SAFE, BE EFFECTIVE, AND GAIN MUSCLE STRENGTH

If you've done any weight lifting, you are familiar with that burning sensation you get in the muscle you're working as you reach the last couple of *repetitions* (often called reps).

To understand why this happens, picture a row of golf clubs (see Figure 2.1).

Opposite the row of clubs is a row of golf balls. Imagine that this row of balls and clubs stretches as far as the eye can see—and beyond. This is your muscle fiber. When your muscle is ready to contract, a sudden chemical reaction occurs, causing an attraction between the clubs and balls. The clubs actually hook onto the balls and pull the line of clubs to the adjacent balls, and the process continues. The clubs and balls represent two proteins that make up your muscle fiber—*actin* (the balls) and *myosin* (the clubs)—and the points at which they make contact are known as *binding sites*.

However, as the muscle continues to contract, lactic acid forms, causing the burning sensation, and this actually inhibits the attraction of golf balls to golf clubs. Imagine a slippery coating forming

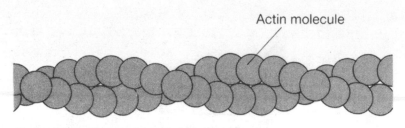

Actin molecule

Actin filament

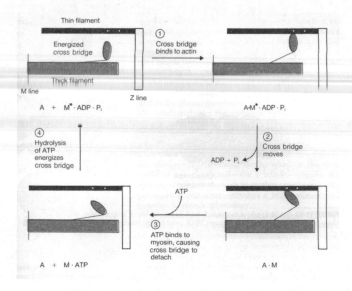

FIGURE 2.1 (a) Two helical chains of actin molecules form the primary structure of the thin filaments; (b) Chemical and mechanical changes during the four stages of a cross-bridge cycle. In a resting muscle fiber, contraction begins with the binding of a cross bridge to actin in a thin filament (step 1).

on the balls so the clubs can't grab onto them to pull themselves along the chain. Eventually, if enough lactic acid builds up, no golf clubs attach to the chain, and the muscle freezes in place — in other words, it cramps. Because no blood can enter a muscle when it contracts, the lactic acid remains in the muscle. Once the contraction ends, the blood supply can continue, and blood helps wash away the built-up lactic acid.

One study (Jun Ding, Anthony S. Wexler, and Stuart A. Binder-Macleod, 2000)[5] has shown that it takes approximately two to two and a half minutes for your blood to wash all the lactic acid from your muscle. When performing a series of *sets* of exercises, if you begin a successive set of reps without waiting for this to occur, then you're not using your entire muscle to lift the weight, and this can lead to a muscle strain. When a client tells me the third set of repetitions is much more difficult than the first, I explain that since the weight is the same, there should be no difference in his or her ability to lift the weight. Once they wait at least two minutes between sets, they realize the effort required is the same as for the first set.

To test this, perform an exercise such as a biceps curl, using a *resistance* that would prevent you from performing an eleventh repetition. Now, wait only ten to twenty seconds, and try to perform ten repetitions. You'll see you can't. Obviously, you didn't get weaker. You simply don't have all the muscle available, because lactic acid has built up, and you didn't wait long enough for it to be removed from the muscle. Now wait two to two and a half minutes, and try again. You'll find you can now perform the set of ten repetitions with the same weight.

The goal of weight training is to make your muscles stronger, allowing you to lift greater and greater amounts of weight. The way this happens is pretty simple. As you apply additional resistance to a muscle, it responds to the increased load by causing *microtears* within the muscle fiber. The body repairs the tears by building more muscle. The muscle fiber thickens and therefore has a greater ability to create force; in effect, the muscle has now gotten stronger. As you continue to increase the load, the fiber continues to thicken, and the muscle continues to get stronger. As long as you continue to increase the load, your body will continue to produce more muscle. Increase your strength by 10 percent, and you have increased your muscle mass by 10 percent. Yet because of the law of diminishing returns, the bigger you get, the more difficult it becomes to add more muscle. Some people call this point a plateau, but there are no plateaus in weight training— just smaller incremental gains that take longer periods of time.

The two types of weight training generally performed are *mass building* and *toning*. Mass building is designed to achieve maximum muscle growth in the shortest period of time. Toning focuses more on the muscle's ability to contract when it's surrounded by lactic acid. Toning is more sports specific, because most sports are performed at such a fast pace that a muscle doesn't have enough time to rest between contractions, which is when the lactic acid could dissipate. Toning helps the muscle achieve maximum strength while still enabling you to perform the sport. Your blood carries lactic acid to the liver, where it's converted to *pyruvic acid*, a substance you can use to create energy. When you tone, you produce more lactic acid in a shorter period of time. As a result, your body adapts by becoming more efficient at removing the lactic acid from the muscle and converting it to pyruvic acid.

You build up lactic acid during sports activities because you're performing in an *anaerobic* state. When you perform an exercise in an *aerobic* capacity, you're taking in a sufficient amount of oxygen. Anaerobic is just the opposite; you're not taking in enough oxygen. This causes lactic acid to develop, triggering the classic feeling of burning in a muscle.

If you're performing mass-building exercises, you'll be able to lift heavier weights than if you're toning. The exercises, however, are exactly the same. The only differences are the number of reps per *set*, or group of reps, and the time you take between sets.

If you're mass building, then the maximum number of reps in a set should be eight. For toning, the maximum number of reps is twelve. To determine the proper weight for the first set, choose a weight that lets you perform the maximum number of repetitions per set comfortably. For the second set, choose a weight that makes it difficult to perform the final rep. For the third and final set, choose a weight that forces you to perform two to three fewer reps than the maximum. As your muscles adapt to the weight, you'll be able to increase the number of reps in the third set. When you reach the maximum and can perform it comfortably, increase the weights for the exercise. That's how you use progressive resistance to get stronger.

When mass building, you perform four to eight repetitions per set, with a two-and-a-half- to three-minute rest interval. Research shows that maximum strength development occurs within four to eight repetitions. If an individual tries to perform fewer than four repetitions in a set, more weight can be used but the chances of performing the technique correctly decreases. This can lead to improper form, overstraining of the affected muscle, and potential injury. Toning calls for ten to twelve repetitions with a thirty-second rest interval. The increased repetition count allows a greater lactic acid buildup to occur while training the muscle to get stronger. The decreased rest interval limits the amount of lactic acid being removed from the muscle. You're performing the exercise with some level of lactic acid in the muscle at all times.

Whether you choose mass building or toning, each triggers an *inflammatory response* to heal the muscle. This, combined with the pain from the microtears, is why your muscles feel sore for a day or two after you lift. Your body releases blood containing healing cells to the injured area, and the increased level of fluid causes swelling. The cells correct the injury, and the swelling disappears.

If the soreness lasts more than two days, you've overtrained the muscle, and you should ease off a little the next session.

When toning, you probably will experience a burning sensation in the muscle. This is just the effect of lactic acid buildup in the muscle. The sensation should dissipate once you complete the set. When mass building, you won't feel this sensation, because the time it takes to complete a set is reduced, so there's not enough time for lactic acid to build up.

Now, let's talk about how to perform an exercise properly. The core idea is that a muscle is put through a full range of motion under a controlled speed with an appropriate resistance. The muscle is shortened and lengthened completely. You shouldn't use *momentum*, and you shouldn't involve any other *muscle groups* other than the one being trained to complete the exercise. If you stick to these guidelines, you'll achieve maximum benefit with the least chance of injury. Contrary to popular belief, most lifting injuries are a result of poor technique, not excessive weight.

Within the bodybuilding community, different fads come and go regarding the most efficient way to manipulate weights to achieve maximum value of time and energy. Most, if not all, of these concepts have no physiological validity and go as fast as they come. They exist solely to fill magazine pages. The better informed you are, the better your chances of achieving your goal, whether it's toning or mass building. Here's a rundown of the different trends, along with their inconsistencies when compared with the basic philosophy of weight training.

Supersetting: When you superset, you complete a set of an exercise and then immediately do another set. Sometimes you do several sets in a row—sometimes with reduced amounts of weights or with different exercises. Some people believe this method is good for mass building or for breaking those so-called plateaus in increasing weights. I disagree.

Supersetting goes against the theory that for the maximum amount of muscle fiber to push the maximum amount of weight, most or all of the lactic acid must be removed from the muscle. If I perform an exercise set with a weight that's so heavy I can complete only eight reps, and then if I immediately do another type of exercise or perform the same exercise with less weight, I haven't fully allowed my bloodstream to remove the lactic acid, not only from the muscles I'm working in the exercise, but also from the stabilizing muscles involved in allowing me to perform the exercise. In fact, I haven't allowed for the lactic acid to be removed at all. The amount of muscle fiber available to lift these weights would be dramatically diminished; I'd feel myself cramping and being able to lift less weight, because I have less muscle fiber available to lift the weight. This goes against the goal of trying to use the greatest amount of muscle fiber to perform an exercise. It does have its merits when conditioning for a particular sport, however, as explained in the section on toning.

The energy source burned while in an aerobic state is fat; for anaerobic, it's carbohydrates. The intensity is what separates aerobic from anaerobic activity. Aerobic exercises are less intense. As the intensity increases, it becomes harder for the body to take in a sufficient amount of oxygen, and the exercise becomes anaerobic. So, even an exercise such as running or jogging, which most people think of as aerobic, can be anaerobic if you're moving at a pace that's fast enough to prevent your body from taking in enough oxygen. Indications that you're in an anaerobic state include burning in a muscle, difficulty speaking while performing the activity, and huffing and puffing.

Because weight training requires a high level of exertion, it's performed in an anaerobic capacity. The only way to make it aerobic would be to lift such an insignificant amount of weight that you'd negate the benefit of the exercise. If you use a sufficient amount of weight to push yourself hard, you'd see that even with a set of six repetitions, you'll be huffing and puffing after the set and will have to stop and catch your breath after the last two sets of any exercise.

Negatives: When you perform the negative element of a set, you perform only the portion of an exercise where the muscle being worked is lengthening. A full range of motion, on the other hand, consists of the muscle shortening and then lengthening. The negative element is an inefficient means of weightlifting. The theory is that a larger percentage of growth occurs during this lengthening period; therefore, it's the only important portion of the repetition. The first problem with this is you now need someone to perform the other half of the repetition while you perform only the negative. You need a spotter for every exercise you perform. This makes you very dependent on others. Second, you lose the joint reception by going through only half the repetition. Your joint receptors send a signal to your brain about how much force is being placed on a joint. Without a full range of motion, your brain sends insufficient nerve signals to the muscle about how much force it has to push against, and an insufficient amount of muscle may be used to lift the weight. Weight training is actually the conditioning of the neurological system. The maximum amount of nerve firing causes the maximum number of muscle fibers to fire. This results in the most efficient lifts and, in turn, the quickest strength gains and subsequent changes in your physique.

Shocking the muscle: Many fitness webzines, magazines, TV shows, and personal trainers argue that if you continue to do the same exercise for a period of time, then a muscle becomes used to the exercise and therefore loses its ability to grow and respond to that exercise. They maintain that you have to redesign your workout at some point, which varies depending on whose opinion you believe. The redesigning could happen every week, month, or in some other time frame. The change can involve going from lighter to heavier weights, exercising different body parts on different days, or totally altering the exercises you perform, thereby shocking the muscle by making it get used to something different. If you understand what's incorporated into a lift, you'll understand why this just can't be correct.

Basically, there are two components to a free-weight lift: balance/stabilization of the weight, and the actual resistance you're lifting. Unlike using weight lifting machines where the motion being performed is set by the machine, free weights (**barbells** or **dumbbells**) move wherever you want—or don't want—them to go. As a result, you must balance and stabilize the free weight, or it will fall. When you begin weight training, you'll be able to increase the amount of resistance very quickly, and progressively it becomes much harder to increase the weight. Obviously, you did not gain any muscle mass in two to three weeks. What's happening initially is that you're expending a tremendous percentage of energy on just balancing and stabilizing the weight and a very small percentage of energy on lifting the resistance. But, as you do it over and over, the body gets used to performing the exercise, and your balance and stabilization improve. You can convert a greater percentage of the energy from balance and stabilization to actually pushing the resistance. With this additional energy, you can now lift more weight. You have in no way altered the amount of muscle fiber available to perform the exercise. You've simply changed the ratio of energy from balance and stabilization to energy spent actually pushing the resistance.

If you can accept this concept, you can now apply it to the idea of shocking the muscle. When you shock a muscle by trying something new, then you're simply diverting most of your energy to the balance and stabilization of the resistance. That's why you'll find that you have to use less weight when you switch exercises or even alter an exercise slightly. Eventually, you get used to the new movement, and you're back where you started, trying to make the muscle adapt to greater and greater amounts of resistance. Ultimately you've delayed your ability to lift heavier weight and grow stronger muscle.

By understanding the physiology of muscle, you'll understand that there are no shortcuts to proper exercise. Weight training takes time. And though it's not something you have to do, it is something you should do to stay healthy and fit as you grow older. It probably won't feel like fun to you. The fun will come in setting goals for yourself and achieving them. Whether for weight loss, battling depression, or general health, weight training will produce a change in your way of life.

3

WHAT IT MEANS WHEN
YOU'RE IN PAIN

Pain in a muscle or joint can be caused by a structural deficit, such as a ***herniated disc*** or arthritis, or a ***mechanical deficit***, such as a muscle weakness. Structural deficits require medical intervention, whereas mechanical deficits can be resolved through strength training. The good news is, in my fifteen years as a physical therapist, I've observed that in 80 to 90 percent of cases I have treated, pain is caused by muscular weakness. This statistic will conflict with statistics from other medical personnel. I want you to hear both sides of the argument and make up your own mind.

A structural cause of pain compromises the tissue's integrity, limiting its ability to function. Examples include a fractured bone, torn ligament, ruptured vertebral disc, and torn cartilage.

Mechanical deficits include muscle weaknesses, muscle imbalances, and flexibility deficits. Muscle imbalances occur when a muscle is stronger than its opposing muscle. Because the stronger muscle has a greater tendency to shorten, it can pull the bone it attaches to out of its proper position, affecting the function of the joint to which it attaches. Shortened muscles can also result from inflammation of a weaker muscle. Let's use the *biceps*, or front upper arm muscle, as an example. The biceps attaches to the upper arm bone, known as the *humerus*. If your biceps is much stronger than your *triceps*, or posterior upper arm muscle, the biceps will shorten, pulling the head of the humerus forward in the shoulder joint. This causes an improper alignment of the humerus and the *glenoid fossa*, or shoulder joint, disrupting normal shoulder function, and can impact tissues at the shoulder joint, causing pain and loss of function.

Classic tests such as x-rays and MRIs look for structural abnormalities that might be causing your pain. But in many cases, the abnormality the doctor finds may have nothing to do with your symptoms. Doctors will often pursue a course of treatment based on the results of x-rays or MRIs, but these tests weren't intended to be the sole means of establishing a diagnosis. A complete clinical evaluation should be performed, with the above tests used to confirm or reject a diagnosis established through the evaluation *Stenosis* of the spine, herniated discs, and arthritis of a joint, for instance, can be indicated by x-rays or MRIs, yet these structural abnormalities might not be the cause of your symptoms.

Most doctors, such as orthopedic surgeons, aren't trained to test for functional limitations; they're trained as surgeons. Muscular deficits won't show up on an MRI or x-ray. The number of patients I've treated who have been diagnosed with structural deficits as the cause of their pain that turn out to be muscular is staggering.

I've treated thousands of patients who've been diagnosed with herniated discs after complaining of pain across the lower back or pain running from the gluteal region or buttocks down the leg. In all but a handful of cases, the cause was muscle *spasms* and weakness. At most, I've seen five or six cases where the symptoms were associated with a herniated disc that impinged on a nerve root.

A herniated disc can't cause pain across the lower back or from the gluteal region down the leg, because there is no nerve pathway through these regions. Yet surgeries are performed to remove parts or whole discs or to fuse the spine in the areas where discs are removed. These surgeries don't address the cause of the symptoms, which is muscle weakness or muscle spasm. In fact, the immobilization required after surgery will likely make their symptoms worse.

One example: a law enforcement agent came to me after a fall that caused pain in his back. He needed to be able to hold a gun up to shoot, but after the fall he was unable to hold his arm up. An orthopedist diagnosed a herniated disc and recommended surgery to relieve the pain in his back and to allow him to regain strength in his arm. I discovered that the fall had caused a *contusion* of the muscles surrounding the right shoulder blade. These muscles hold the shoulder blade against the ribs when you lift your arm. If they're weak, you can't hold your arm up. After two weeks of treatment, his symptoms were resolved.

Carpal tunnel syndrome is another often misdiagnosed injury. People have come to me after an *electromyography* (EMG) indicated that they had this condition. In some cases, the doctor recommended physical therapy rather than surgery; in others, the patients came to me on their own. They complained of numbness in all their fingers, even though carpal tunnel syndrome, which relates to compression of the *median nerve*, affects only the thumb, index finger, middle finger, and half of the ring finger. In each of these cases, the decreased nerve conduction speed that the diagnostic test revealed may have existed, but this was not what was causing the symptoms.

Many patients have come to me after doctors told them that the cause of their pain or dysfunction was structural. They resorted to medication over extensive periods of time, without relief. In most cases, their doctors didn't change the treatment protocol because the diagnosis called for medication or surgery, and the patients were unwilling to accept surgery as an option. Those who did resort to surgery found that their symptoms remained. The structural variation was there, but that's not what was causing their symptoms.

These people eventually accepted living with pain on a daily basis, assuming there were no alternatives. Typically, through recommendations from others I've treated, they ended up at my facility. In most cases, I found the cause of their problems to be weak muscles or muscle imbalances affecting the performance of the muscle or joint in question. With basic heat and massage, followed by stretching and aggressive strength training, the symptoms disappeared, and these individuals went on to live pain-free lives.

Even people who do have structural problems—a herniated disc, shrinkage of a joint space at the knee, or arthritis in a joint—can return to proper function without drugs or surgery. In most cases, the joint will function well. In fact, a joint's health and capacity is more about the strength, flexibility, and balance of the surrounding musculature than it is about the joint's structural components. Many of my patients have fully resolved their pain, loss of range of motion, and decreased functional capacity through strength training, despite having herniated discs, arthritis in a joint, or shrinkage of a joint space. X-rays or MRIs taken before and after the symptoms were resolved probably would look the same.

Once I'm able to determine that the cause of a symptom is mechanical, I can help build a patient's strength and very quickly resolve the symptom. Many patients jokingly call it a "miracle" when they limp in and walk out or when they raise an arm over their head and they couldn't before. But it's no miracle; it's just a matter of understanding how a joint functions and fixing what caused it to break down. In a substantial number of patients I've treated, the cause of the dysfunction was mechanical (muscular) in nature, so they were able to overcome problems through strength training even if a structural deficit was present. Certainly, I've had cases where a structural deficit *was* the cause of the individual's dysfunction, and, in those cases, I referred the patient to proper medical personnel for treatment.

Medical research (Monica J. Daley and Warwick L. Spinks, 2000)[2] now confirms that proper strength training can help limit, if not prevent, the typical causes of daily dysfunction. Besides keeping muscles strong and joints stable, strength training increases *venous flow*, limiting the effects of many cardiovascular diseases. It also increases bone density and reduces the risk of osteoporosis and bone fractures. If there's swelling in a region of the body, such as a hand or foot, strength training increases the contractile force of the muscles in the region, enhancing the lymphatic system's ability to remove the swelling. The lymphatic system helps keep the area between cells free of contaminants such as bacteria.

Another secret of strength training is that it increases the body's resting metabolic rate, increasing the need to burn fat at all times, even at rest. Altering your resting metabolic rate is the quickest and most efficient way to burn fat and decrease fat deposits in the body.

I believe strength training is often the only way to resolve symptoms such as pain or loss of range of motion at a joint regardless of whether medical attention is sought. Strength training also can prevent most of the symptoms associated with overuse injuries, or in many cases, lack-of-use injuries such as back strains and knee pain. When evaluating someone for the first time, there are questions I need to ask to draw a conclusion about the cause of the symptoms. The answers to these five questions help me determine whether symptoms at a joint are caused by a mechanical or by a structural deficit(s):

1. *What is the mechanism of injury, or what brought on the symptom in the first place?* Was it a traumatic injury such as a fall or an impact from an object? Was it a repetitive type of injury resulting from playing a sport or repeated use of a tool, a computer, or other work equipment? Did the symptom peak suddenly, or did it progress slowly? If the symptom results from a specific activity, often that symptom is muscular in nature and can be resolved through

strength training. If it stems from a traumatic incident such as a car accident, a fall, or an impact injury, it's more likely structural and will probably require some form of medical treatment.

2. *Does activity lessen or worsen the severity of the symptom?* If you have back pain, for instance, and walking makes the pain decrease, then the cause is probably muscular in nature. Walking heats up the muscles of the lower back, causing them to relax, which reduces pain. If the cause is a fractured vertebra or a herniated disc pressing on another tissue, then walking would aggravate the situation.

3. *How much range of motion, both passive and active, is present at the joint?* Active refers to the range of motion an individual can create when moving a joint on his own. Passive refers to the degree to which someone else can move the joint without the person's assistance. If active range of motion is limited while passive is full, the cause of the symptom is most likely muscular and can be resolved through exercise. If both are limited, the cause of the symptom is probably structural and will require medical intervention.

As an example, let's use biceps **tendonitis** versus severe arthritis of the shoulder. If you have biceps tendonitis, you'd have decreased active range of motion because it takes muscle to move the joint on its own. But with **passive range of motion**, you'd feel no pain, because someone else moving your joint would require no muscular contraction on your part. Because there's nothing structurally wrong with the joint, you'd have full passive shoulder motion with tendonitis.

Now, let's look at a shoulder with severe arthritis. In this case, both the active and passive ranges of motion would be limited, because the arthritic change limits the space in the joint, preventing normal motion. Even if you had full strength, neither you nor someone else would be able to move the joint through full range of motion. Range of motion is one of the most critical elements in determining if a symptom is structural or mechanical. I've had patients who were diagnosed with arthritis of the shoulder but had full passive range of motion. What does this tell you about their shoulders? It indicates that although some arthritic change has occurred, the cause of the symptom is still mechanical, not structural, and strengthening can resolve it.

This is one of the areas I spend the most time explaining to patients. Although diagnostic testing reveals conditions such as arthritis, **bone spurs**, and herniated discs, these conditions may be *benign* and have no bearing on function. You must conduct further tests, such as the ones I describe, to determine whether these structural abnormalities require treatment or are irrelevant.

4. *If you touch the area, what type of tissue is irritated or inflamed?* When people experience pain, particularly in the neck and lower back, it's often mistakenly diagnosed as structural. Diagnoses include herniated discs, stenosis, and arthritis of the spine. But if any of these are the cause of the symptoms, the pain would be at the spine where the herniated disc, stenosis, or arthritis is identified. In a majority of the cases I've seen, patients felt the pain across their lower backs several inches away from the spine. This is where the lower back muscles are, indicating that the cause of the symptoms is muscular and that proper strengthening exercises could resolve the symptoms.

5. *What is the type and severity of the symptom?* Obviously, if a symptom is severe, it must be taken more seriously than a less intense symptom, and constant symptoms are always more of a concern than intermittent ones. One of the biggest clues to the cause of a symptom is whether it's highly definable in a specific area or hard to pinpoint. If it's definable, the tissue being touched is the inflamed tissue, and that's what you need to address. If it's hard to pinpoint, then a tissue in another area is causing the symptom. This is called a **referred** symptom. The most obvious example relates to the heart. One of the signs of heart difficulties is a diffuse, nonspecific pain down the left arm. Clearly nothing is wrong

with your left arm, but that's where you're feeling the pain. You may even say you have the symptom but can't pinpoint its location. The same holds true for muscles and nerves, both of which can refer symptoms to specific locations based on the wiring of the body. As mentioned earlier, numbness at the thumb, index finger, middle finger, and half the ring finger can indicate some form of compression of the median nerve—a condition known as carpal tunnel syndrome. Numbness in all the fingers can be a referred sensation from the **rotator cuff**, located at the shoulder. To zero in on the true cause of the symptom and determine whether exercise can resolve the symptom, you need to answer all the questions above. You can use diagnostic testing afterward to confirm or reject the potential cause.

I'm not dismissing the need for medical attention. I'm trying to give you a better understanding of the human body and provide a very conservative approach to resolving some of the basic causes of symptoms that plague people on a daily basis. In my experience, in most cases, these symptoms are caused by lack of proper fitness and can be resolved in a few weeks. If they're not cured by strength training, medical attention is still available, and waiting several weeks to start a medication or have surgery won't usually worsen your symptoms. If exercise is performed correctly, the exercise will not increase symptoms, even if the cause of the symptoms is structural. Everything described in this book is based on my fifteen years of experience treating patients with pain, loss of range of motion at a joint, swelling at a joint, or altered sensations such as tingling, burning, numbness, or weakness. Aside from basic care such as moist heat, massage, and other forms of treatment, strength training ultimately resolved their symptoms and returned them to pain-free, fully functional lives.

The following is a rundown of common areas of pain, information on determining whether the cause is muscular, and if it is, the muscles you should strengthen to relieve the symptoms.

The Neck

*Muscles to strengthen to resolve neck symptoms include
the posterior deltoids (pg. 139), interscapular muscles,
including the mid-traps and rhomboids (pg. 90), triceps
(posterior upper arm muscles)(pg. 141), and rotator cuff
(pg. 141).*

Very few of the neck complaints I've seen have actually been associated directly with the neck, and those were due to severe cases of
arthritis. Most of my patients diagnosed with neck arthritis didn't
have a significant enough degree of arthritis to create the symptoms they described. Instead, a muscle imbalance was causing the
symptoms. After completing strength training, their symptoms resolved, even with the arthritis.

In addition to arthritis, common diagnoses of the neck include
herniated discs and stenosis of the spine. Yet, for these diagnoses to
be correct, the area of pain would have to be strictly at the spine
and only in the immediate area of the structural deficit. If your
pain is in the skull, neck, or from the neck down to the shoulder,
then a diagnosis of herniated disc or stenosis is inaccurate.

In the case of a herniated disc, the disc itself can't be painful, because there's no nerve supply at the disc. For you to feel pain, the
disc has to press on an adjacent tissue. If it presses on the tissues that
surround the spinal cord to provide stability, you'd expect to feel pain
running up and down the spine, but only at the spine. If the disc
impinged on a nerve root (nerve roots come out of the spinal cord
at every level of the spine and innervate certain muscles and certain
areas of skin), you'd expect to have symptoms associated only with the
innervated muscle and area of skin innervated by that vertebral level.

I've had no more than a handful of patients with a diagnosis of
herniated disc who actually displayed some form of the symptoms
associated with this condition. A study in the *New England Journal of*

Medicine (Maureen C. Jensen, Michael N. Brant-Zawadzki, Nancy Obuchowski, Michael T. Modic, Dennis Malkasian, and Jeffrey S. Ross, 1994)[7] showed that almost 70 percent of the population has some form of herniated or bulging discs without symptoms. The study concluded that the discovery by MRI of bulges or protrusions in people with low back pain frequently is coincidental.

In the case of spinal stenosis, the vertebrae move closer together because the space between them shrinks. The biggest loss of range of motion occurs during extension, when tilting your head up. Other motions, such as looking side to side or bringing your ear to your shoulder, are unaffected. Most of the patients I've treated have had a limited ability to move their heads up, down, or from side to side. To some degree, most also had difficulty rotating their heads.

Symptoms associated with the neck are actually more a shoulder and shoulder blade issue than a neck issue. Most neck pain and headaches are the result of strength imbalance between the muscles of the front upper arm (biceps), front torso (pectoral), and front shoulder (anterior deltoid) and those of the posterior upper arm (triceps), posterior torso, and posterior shoulder. Typically, the muscles in the front are stronger than those in the back, because for most of the activities we perform, we use the front of the body—whether it's lifting, holding, or moving an object. Naturally, the muscle that's in the best position to create force when performing an activity is the one you'll use.

Due to this muscle imbalance, the muscles used more often have a tendency to shorten. Because of their attachment to the shoulder blade, the shortening causes the shoulder blade to move outward away from the spine. The shoulder joint is created by the upper arm bone and the end of the shoulder blade. As the shoulder joint is drawn forward, the inner border of the shoulder blade moves away from the spine. As this happens, any muscle that attaches from the skull or the spine to the shoulder blade is overstretched and is more susceptible to pain and inflammation.

Overstretched muscles also lose their ability to create force and support the head or stabilize the shoulder blade to allow for normal shoulder function. This is a result of the muscles breaking down and becoming inflamed. Based on their attachment to the skull and cervical spine, they can limit neck motion, making it appear as if the cause of the symptoms is neck related.

Because of their attachment to multiple neck vertebrae, these muscles may cause the vertebrae to be pulled together. As this happens, a vacuum seal may form between them. Imagine turning an empty coffee cup with a wet rim upside down on a counter. A seal forms between the cup and the counter, and you'll find it difficult to lift the cup. As you force the cup off the counter, you'll usually hear a popping sound, that's the vacuum seal breaking. It's the same with the neck. The vacuum seal prevents you from moving your neck from side to side or up and down. If you try to move your neck quickly, you may hear a popping sound, and suddenly you'll be able to move your neck with greater ease. You just broke the vacuum seal at the neck vertebrae, allowing for freer motion. The problem is that if you don't resolve the tightening of the surrounding muscles by correcting the muscle strength imbalance, then the vacuum seal will continue to form. This seal prevents the vertebrae from gliding properly, and you'll continue to have pain and decreased range of motion at the neck joints. What's more, if you have arthritis and you don't maintain proper gliding of the vertebral bodies, the arthritis could worsen.

People with this type of muscle-strength imbalance often complain of chronic headaches, because the muscles that attach to the skull are tightening up and pulling on the skull.

The Lower Back

To maintain a healthy lower back, you need to strengthen your glutes (pg. 114, st. leg deadlifts), hamstrings (pg.

112), *hip abductors (pg. 118), and abdominals (pg. 77, trunk curl).*

No area of the body is affected by other parts of the body as much as the lower back. Common diagnoses of this region are similar to those for the neck, with arthritis, herniated discs, and spinal stenosis the most common. As with the neck, in cases where the patient has been diagnosed with arthritis, I've seen few instances where the symptoms were actually the result of the arthritic changes. In most cases, arthritic changes occur with little or no effect on joint function.

Herniated discs are a common diagnosis in cases where symptoms include pain, numbness, or tingling in the lower extremities. As mentioned earlier, a herniated disc alone can't cause pain, because there's no nerve supply in the disc. The lower back, or lumbar region, of the spine has five vertebrae, numbered L1 through L5. If a herniated disc were impinging a nerve root at L3, you may feel an altered sensation at the front of your thigh and note weakness only of the muscle at that location. If a herniated disc was impinging a bit lower, at L4, you'd feel an altered sensation at the inside portion of the shin, and it would prevent the **anterior tibialis** (the muscle that raises the ankle toward the face) from functioning properly.

In almost all cases I've seen in which an individual was diagnosed with a herniated disc, the symptoms began in the gluteal region and ran down the side of the thigh and lower leg or the back of the thigh and lower leg and sometimes all the way down to the foot. These symptoms aren't indicative of a herniated disc; they're indicative of a syndrome known as sciatica. Sciatica usually results from an inflammation of the sciatic nerve as it passes through the gluteal region and becomes impinged on by the **piriformis** muscle. The piriformis muscle runs across the gluteal region and has a tendency to become inflamed and impinge on the sciatic nerve when other muscles in the pelvic or torso regions are weak and unable to perform their functions.

The diagnosis of spinal stenosis makes sense only if the greatest loss of range of motion occurs while leaning backward, because as the space between the vertebrae decreases, the vertebrae get closer together and sometimes even touch. In the neck and lower back region, the backs of the vertebrae are closer together because of the natural arch in the spine. This causes an inability to bend backward. The majority of the patients I've treated who've been diagnosed with spinal stenosis have been limited primarily in bending forward and then in side-to-side movement and rotation.

In most cases I've seen with neck and lower back pain, the symptoms have resulted from weakness or muscle imbalances of the upper and lower extremities. Weaknesses and imbalances can leave the lower back overworked or fixed in an improper position, causing severe pain and limiting all functional capacity. I've had patients whose back pain prevented them from standing erect or walking without a cane. Naturally, they thought something terrible had to be wrong. In most cases, however, it was just a muscle-strength imbalance between the front and posterior hip and thigh muscles.

The most common muscle-strength imbalance is between the hip flexors (front hip muscles) and quads (quadriceps) and the muscles of the gluteus region (buttocks) and the hamstrings (posterior thigh muscles). Everyday movements, including walking, standing, climbing stairs, sitting down, or standing up, require contractions of the hip flexor and quads. When you're walking, the quadriceps create the kick to move the leg forward to make the step, while the hamstrings work to slow the leg down, stop, and prepare it for landing the foot to support you again.

Most people's quads and hip flexors are much stronger than their glutes and hamstrings. As a result, the quads tend to shorten, and because the quads attach to the front of the pelvis, the shortening pulls the front of the pelvis down. This is called an ***anterior tilt***. As this occurs, the back of the pelvis rises, moving closer to the rib cage, increasing the arch at the lower back. The main lower back muscles attach from the lower ribs to the top of the pelvis. When the distance between these two landmarks shortens, the muscles shorten, making them susceptible to spasm. This spasm limits any motion of the lower back and inhibits ability to support your body weight. In certain cases, the spasm is on only one side, forcing your body to curve sideways, and you'll appear as if you're falling to one side.

To resolve this situation, limit the shortening of the quads and hip flexors by strengthening your glutes and hamstrings. Once you do, the front of your pelvis won't be pulled down, the back of the pelvis won't be pulled up, your lower back muscles won't shorten, and you limit your chance of going into spasm.

Many people are under the mistaken impression that weak lower back muscles are the cause of pain in the lower back. This is only true if an individual has been bedridden for an extensive period of time. If maintained at a proper length through proper strengthening of the thigh and glute muscles, the lower back muscles are more than adequate to support the upper torso weight and even assist in lifting if you don't employ perfect mechanics (squatting down to lift and keeping your shoulders, knees, and ankles in alignment). Lower back muscles break down and create such severe pain because their length is compromised due to an improper position of the pelvis caused by muscle-strength imbalances.

Strengthening your abdominals is not the primary means of maintaining a pain-free back either. The ***abdominal sheath*** is fairly thin, and due to its attachment from ribs and sternum to the pelvis, it's not in a good position to create force. The main purpose of the abdominal muscle group is to maintain the abdominal wall in support of your visceral organs, because there's no skeletal support in this region.

Another misconception is that obesity is the main cause of lower back pain. Although it is a contributing factor, it's not the primary cause. If it were, then the only way to resolve the pain would be to lose weight. I've had morbidly obese patients who resolved their lower back pain not by losing weight but by correcting the muscle-strength imbalance. Certainly, losing weight if you're obese will decrease the stresses put on your lower back, just as strengthening your abdominals will help offset the severe strength deficit between the lower back muscles and abdominals and will help pull in the girth in the abdominal region. But there's nothing more effective in resolving most cases of lower back pain than achieving a proper muscle balance between the hip flexors and quads versus the hamstrings and glutes. More than anything else, this will help you maintain your lower back muscles at their proper length, allowing for proper force output of these muscles.

The hip *abductor* muscles also help you maintain proper length of the lower back muscles. These are the muscles on the sides of the hips that help to stabilize the pelvis when balancing your weight on a single leg—something you do every time you take a step. There's a strong correlation between weak hip abductors and inflamed lower-back muscles. The torso stabilizers, including your lower back muscles and your hip stabilizers—most importantly the hip abductors—work in conjunction with one another. If one group is weak, it can cause the other group to break down and become inflamed. This is more common when an individual complains of lower back pain on only one side.

The Shoulder

The muscles to strengthen to maintain a healthy shoulder are the posterior deltoids (pg. 139), rhomboids and mid-traps (pg. 90), triceps (pg. 141), and rotator cuff (pg. 141). If no symptoms exist, you can also work on the entire deltoid group (pg. 132, military press), the biceps (pg. 100, bicep curl), and the upper traps (pg. 139, shrugs).

When someone complains of shoulder pain, the diagnosis is often arthritis. Although it can be found on an x-ray, arthritis is a factor in the pain only if both an individual's active and passive range of motion are affected. I've treated many patients with shoulder pain who were diagnosed with arthritis of the shoulder yet achieved full pain-free active and passive range of motion after treatment. This is because the arthritis was not causing the pain; it was a muscle-strength imbalance. Bone spurs also fall into the category of arthritis. These calcium deposits can develop under the shoulder bone (under the *acromium process*). If the deposit is large enough, it will affect the space between the arm bone and the shoulder bone. As you raise your arm over shoulder height, the space between the arm bone and shoulder bone becomes smaller, increasing the chance of impingement on the tendons or *bursae* in the area. A bursa is a purse of fluid that sits between two tissues to prevent friction and pain. Again, a simple x-ray is not a determining factor, because the x-ray identifies only the bone spur and not a possible strain. Loss of passive range of motion must exist to confirm that a bone spur is the cause of shoulder pain.

Another case of shoulder pain is "frozen shoulder" (adhesive capsulitis), a situation where the joint capsule that surrounds the shoulder, which is typically very lax to allow for severe range of motion, becomes inflamed and loses its elasticity. As a result, both active and passive ranges of motion are lost. Whether the cause of pain is arthritis or frozen shoulder, physical therapy or treatment from a physician is needed.

If the cause of pain or loss of active range of motion is a muscular weakness or an imbalance causing the joint to act improperly and irritate the tissues, strength training is the only solution. In most of these cases, the muscles of the front torso, shoulder, and upper arm are stronger than their posterior counterparts, creating a condition referred to as forward shoulder posture. This imbalance pulls the humeral head forward toward the front of the joint and overstretches the biceps muscle, which travels around the head of the humerus to attach at the top of the shoulder joint. With the humeral head pulled forward in the shoulder joint, there's a greater possibility it will impinge on or compress the muscles between the humeral head and the acromium process: the biceps, *supraspinatus*, and *infraspinatus*.

The other tissue in the space beneath the acromium process (the subacromial space) is the ***subacromial bursa***. The subacromial bursa also can become injured as a result of the humeral head being pulled forward. Most cases of nontraumatic tendonitis and bursitis are caused by this muscle imbalance. The main clinical finding necessary to denote bursitis as the cause of pain at the shoulder is swelling noted just in front of the bone that sits on top of the shoulder joint. I have never seen this, leaving me to conclude that the diagnosis of bursitis is incorrectly given in many cases.

The other key to the functional capacity of the shoulder joint is the rotator cuff. Consisting of four muscles that attach from and around the shoulder blade to the humeral head, the rotator cuff's main function is to prevent the humeral head from rising into the acromium process when you lift your arm over shoulder height. This is depressing the head of the humerus. If your rotator cuff is weak, the humeral head will rise and impinge on the tendons and bursae that sit between the humeral head and the acromium process. If you maintain the proper muscle balance between the muscles of the anterior shoulder, pecs (chest), and biceps, and those of the posterior shoulder, upper back, and triceps, and you maintain proper strength of the rotator cuff, the shoulder joint will function optimally, limiting the chance of injury.

The Elbow

The muscles to strengthen to achieve full function of the elbow are the triceps (pg. 141), biceps (pg. 100), wrist flexors (pg. 106, wrist curl), and wrist extensors (pg. 106, wrist curl for extension).

The muscles that relate to the elbow are those of the forearm—the wrist flexors and extensors. These muscles attach to the elbow, but their function is to bend the wrist toward the palm (wrist flexion) or toward the back of the hand (wrist extension). If an inflammation is of the wrist extensors, it's commonly known as tennis elbow (lateral epicondylitis); if it's of the wrist flexors, it's known as golfer's elbow (medial epicondylitis). Tennis elbow results from weakened wrist extensors and causes pain at the outside of the elbow, loss of range of motion of the wrist, and weakness and pain when trying to hold an object. Symptoms of golfer's elbow include pain at the inside of the elbow, loss of range of motion at the wrist when flexing the wrist downward, difficulty lifting objects with the affected arm, and weakness at the forearm.

The elbow joint itself is a simple hinge joint, so it only bends and extends. Thus, very little mobility is achieved at this joint. The biceps attaches to the front of the elbow and the triceps attaches to the back of the elbow. These muscles typically aren't injured other than in traumatic incidents. That's why elbow pain is rarely injured experienced other than in traumatic incidents or as a result of the overuse syndromes of tennis elbow or golfer's elbow.

My biggest concern regarding common treatment of these two syndromes is when a physician immediately uses cortisone. No attempt is made to resolve the condition by achieving muscle balance through strengthening both muscle groups so the patient can accomplish the activity or task that created the breakdown in the first place. Cortisone shots never resolve the cause of symptoms; they simply limit the symptom in an area. They also limit the patient's ability to determine if further damage is occurring when the same activity or task that initiated the symptoms is attempted. The goal of any treatment, including strength training, should be to resolve the cause of the symptoms to prevent them from reoccurring, not to simply mask the symptoms. Strength training achieves this goal.

To resolve tennis elbow, you need to strengthen the wrist extensors—unless it's shortened as a result of being inflamed. To see whether this is the case, keep your elbow locked (straight) and use your other hand to bend the affected arm's wrist forward. Now do the same with your other wrist. If the affected wrist doesn't bend as far as the other wrist, then don't strengthen the wrist extensors yet. Just strengthen the wrist flexors until you can stretch the extensors as far as the unaffected wrist's extensors. Once you can do this, you can strengthen the wrist extensors until you obtain maximum strength and functional capacity.

In most of the cases of golfer's elbow I've treated, the patient's wrist flexors were stronger than his or her wrist extensors This is a common muscle imbalance. When wrist extensors are much weaker than wrist flexors, the wrist flexors shorten and become inflamed and painful. The **length-tension ratio** states that a muscle that's shortened or overstretched loses its ability to create force. The reason for the decreased force output is because at the shortened or lengthened state, there is decreased cross bridging of the actin and myosin fibers. A muscle that's stronger than its opposing muscle will shorten, and as it does, there are fewer binding sites where the two proteins that make up muscle fibers can join to create force. As a result, the muscle will appear weaker in the shortened position. Only at its normal length can it create optimum strength and perform its function most effectively.

The Wrist

The muscles to strengthen to maintain a healthy wrist joint and achieve full functional capacity of the wrist include the wrist flexors (pg. 106, wrist curl) and extensors (pg. 106, wrist curl for extension).

The most common diagnosis associated with wrist symptoms is carpal tunnel syndrome. Physicians often attribute symptoms such as tingling, numbness, burning, or pain to carpal tunnel syndrome when the cause may not be related to that condition. Most of my patients who complain of numbness or altered sensation in their hands say it affects all their fingers. Carpal tunnel syndrome describes inflammation of the muscles and tendons of the finger flexors (the muscles that close your fingers), which ultimately impinge on the median nerve as they pass through the carpal tunnel (the space between the wrist or carpal bones and the flexor *retinaculum*, or connective tissue band, that holds the tendons described in place). As mentioned earlier, compression of the median nerve will send altered sensations only to the thumb, index finger, middle finger, and half the ring finger, so if your symptoms are at all the fingers, then compression of the median nerve can't be the cause.

A positive EMG test can indicate slow conduction speed of the median nerve, but a slower nerve conduction speed in this hand may be normal for you—and not what's causing the symptoms. The only real way of knowing if this is a factor in what's causing the problem is if you'd had the test before the symptoms arose. Unless a previous test indicated a faster speed before symptoms, the test is inconclusive. Other issues besides carpal tunnel syndrome can cause altered sensations in the hand, and the specific type and location of the symptom can help determine what's causing the problem.

It's also important to address the mechanism of injury that may have caused what's known as referred symptoms to the hand. Let's say you noticed a tingling or numbness in your hand after waking up in the morning. You also have pain in your neck on the same side as the numb hand, and you recall having had a difficult night's sleep, during which you tossed and turned. You're now finding it difficult to rotate your head or bend it to the side, and your neck muscles are in spasm. What happened was that you slept with your head in an awkward position, causing your neck muscles to become inflamed and thickened after being in a shortened position. They're pressing on the nerves that go through the **upper trapezius** (trap) region of the neck under the collarbone. These nerves go down to the hand. This is where the referred symptoms are coming from. To correct these symptoms, you'd need to relax the neck muscles to take pressure off the impinged nerves.

Altered sensations in the hand can also derive from the rotator cuff. When inflamed, the muscles of the rotator cuff can refer symptoms to the hand. If you performed an activity of a repetitive nature for an extended period of time and noticed sore back and shoulder muscles in conjunction with numbness in your hand, there's a good chance the numbness is coming from an inflamed rotator cuff. To resolve these symptoms, your rotator cuff muscles would have to be treated to eliminate the inflammation.

There are many causes of referred symptoms in the hand or fingers. In the cases I've described, appropriate strengthening of the muscles creating the symptoms might resolve the problems without further treatment.

If you're diagnosed with carpal tunnel syndrome, have the associated symptoms, and can establish a cause associated with straining the wrist or finger flexors (the muscles on top of your forearm, which bend your wrist toward your palm), the way to resolve the symptoms is to reduce the inflammation of these muscles.

Many believe that surgery is the only alternative. To appreciate why this is not the case, you need to understand what causes carpal tunnel syndrome. Overuse and repetitive activities can cause the wrist and finger flexors and their tendons to become inflamed. Because the carpal tunnel has very little ability to accept the swelling of the tendons, the median nerve that also passes through the tunnel becomes compressed, causing symptoms. The surgery involves putting a slit in the retinaculum (the thick connective tissue band that forms the carpal tunnel) to allow it to expand for the increased area requirement of the inflamed tendons. The forearm is immobilized while healing takes place, and scar tissue develops at the incision site. Unfortunately, the

scar tissue causes the retinaculum to become more rigid and therefore incapable of expanding to accommodate an inflamed tendon.
When you return to the activity that caused the inflammation, it will
recur, because you still haven't conditioned those muscles and tendons to be able to perform the activity. The very symptoms the surgery
was supposed to eliminate will be back.

The solution is to condition the muscles and tendons to handle
the stress that the repetitive activity places on them. If an activity causes an area of the body to break down, it's an indication
that the muscles are unprepared to accomplish the activity. You
have two ways to solve the problem: stop performing the activity
or condition yourself to perform it without causing inflammation.
Most people don't think twice about conditioning themselves for
a sport, but conditioning themselves to type or clean the house is
a foreign concept. If you perform an activity on a repetitive basis,
you must strengthen the muscles you use to perform it to accept
the additional stress. This is why everyone should perform some
form of overall strength training. If the entire body is strong and
ready to perform any activity, even a repetitive one, you drastically
reduce your chances of injury.

In most cases, carpal tunnel syndrome is caused by a muscle
imbalance between the wrist or finger flexors and extensors. The
wrist flexors are usually much stronger than the extensors, and, as
a result, they shorten and lose their ability to create force. When
this happens, they can't perform the function they need to perform, and they break down. To begin to resolve the symptoms,
strengthen the wrist extensors. Once you can bend your wrist back
toward the top of your forearm to the same degree that you can
bend your unaffected wrist, you can begin strengthening the wrist
flexors. Your goal, as always, is to keep the wrist flexors and extensors balanced so neither will have a tendency to shorten. Strong,
flexible, balanced muscles produce the maximum output and limit the chance of injury.

Another diagnosis at the wrist and hand is arthritis. As with other areas of the body, the degree of arthritis might not affect the functional capacity of the joint. I've frequently seen a severe shortening of the flexor or extensor tendons that pass across the wrist to the hands and fingers. The shortening of these tendons causes increased compression of the bony surfaces of the joints, creating vacuum seals. This reduces the motion at the joints and increases the amount of joint surface rubbing. That's what causes the pain. In most of these cases, strengthening exercises resolves the shortening of the muscles in the forearm, which also prevents shortening of the tendons that lead to the wrist and fingers. This takes pressure off the joints by limiting surface tension. The reduced friction of the joint surfaces limits joint pain

The Hip

The muscles to strengthen to maintain a healthy hip include the gluteus maximus (pg. 114, st. leg deadlifts), hamstrings (pg. 112), hip abductors (pg. 118), and hip adductors (pg. 120). You should strengthen the hip adductors only after you've strengthened the hip abductors to the point where you can use the same amount of weight for both.

The most common diagnoses of structural abnormalities of the hip region are arthritis and trochanteric **bursitis**. The **trochanteric bursa** sits between the **femur** (thighbone) and the skin. It allows for normal hip function by preventing the irritation of two tissues coming in contact with each other.

One of the key ways to differentiate these two diagnoses from a strained muscle is to press on the painful area. With trochanteric bursitis, your hip joint would be painful, because the bursa sits just superficial to it. The area around your hip joint would be swollen because of increased fluid in the bursa sac, but it would not be painful to the touch. In the case of arthritis, the pain would be only at the joint itself and not in the surrounding tissue. With arthritis, you would suffer a severe loss of both active and passive range of motion. You may find that, as the joint is put through its range of motion, it feels as if it gets caught and then releases a bit further and gets caught again and releases further still and so on.

Another symptom associated with hip arthritis is a referred pain in the groin region. This is not exclusively the result of hip arthritis. If one of the muscles that attaches to the hip joint becomes inflamed and shortens, the femur can be compressed into the hip socket with great force, causing the joint surfaces to rub with greater friction. The surfaces will become irritated and create the referred groin pain. So just because you have groin pain doesn't mean you have arthritis of the hip. If one of the muscles around the hip is inflamed, painful to touch, and weak, this is more likely to be the cause of the groin pain. An x-ray or MRI should not be the determining factor in diagnosing the cause of hip symptoms. A complete evaluation of the surrounding tissue must be conducted to make a correct diagnosis and determine the proper treatment protocol.

Strength training can resolve symptoms if the muscles that surround the hip have become weak. The hip joint comprises the femur and the pelvic bone (acetabulum), so the muscles that attach to these bones—the piriformis and the gluteus medius (hip abductors)—affect the joint's health. The piriformis attaches from the sacral spine (the lowest portion of the spine) to the greater trochanter (a protuberance near the neck of the femur). The piriformis sits even deeper in the gluteal region than the gluteus maximus (the buttocks muscles) and will become inflamed when the other muscles in the pelvic region are weak and can't assist it in supporting a person's body weight. This can cause pain at the gluteal region or can impinge on the sciatic nerve, which can refer pain or tingling down the side or back of the leg as far down as the foot. This is called sciatica.

Even though the piriformis is inflamed and providing the symptom, it's the weakening of other muscles such as the gluteus maximus, gluteus medius, and hamstrings (posterior thigh muscles) that have caused the piriformis to become inflamed. In most of the cases I've seen, the weakness is at the gluteus maximus and gluteus medius. The gluteus medius can become weak if an individual walks or stands for prolonged periods.

The gluteus medius muscles sit on the outside of the pelvic region, just above the hip joint. Their purpose is to keep the pelvis level while walking or running, when a person has to balance on one leg while swinging the other. As you swing your leg, your foot passes just above the ground. If the gluteus medius muscles on the standing leg are weak, the opposite hip will drop, and you might find yourself tripping often or catching your foot on the ground when walking. Many patients who have this problem think they are just clumsy.

As with any activity that you're performing frequently or for a long duration, you need to condition the muscles involved to perform the task without breaking down. I've found a strong correlation between weak gluteus medius or maximus muscles and an inflamed piriformis. Your hips support a substantial amount of your body weight. You need to strengthen these muscles appropriately to prevent symptoms or dysfunction.

Another issue to discuss is the possibility of a muscle imbalance at the hip, resulting from the hip flexors being much stronger than the hip extensors. The hip flexors include two muscles, the iliacus and the psoas, which attach at the inner pelvic region and the lumbar spine, respectively. They're joined by a common tendon at the femur, near the hip joint. The hip extensors include the gluteus maximus and the hamstrings. As noted, it's not uncommon for the hip extensors to be weak due to a lack of hip extension in normal daily function. As a result, the hip flexors will be stronger than the hip extensors, causing the flexors to shorten. In shortening, they pull on the lumbar spine, creating an increased arching. This can cause the muscles that attach in this area to shorten and be susceptible to spasm. This is another situation where the symptom is in one location and its cause is in another.

The **adductors** attach from the pelvic bone to different areas along the femur all the way down to the knee. Because this attachment extends so far down the femur, these muscles have a tremendous ability to create force. This is in stark contrast to the hip abductors, which include one muscle that attaches from the pelvis to the hip joint and another that consists mostly of connective tissue attaching to the knee joint. The hip abductors have a greater tendency to be weak, so if you strengthen the hip adductors without equally strengthening the hip abductors, the adductors will shorten and become susceptible to straining or tearing. Women are often told they need to strengthen their hip adductor muscles to avoid fat deposits in the inner thigh area and have a more shapely leg. But strengthening all the muscles of the body will increase its need to burn fat, including the fat at the inner thigh.

The Knee

The muscles to strengthen to maintain a healthy knee include the quads (pg. 108, squats, and pg. 114, leg press), hamstrings (pg. 112), calf (gastrocnemius aspect) (pg. 126, donkey calf raise), hip abductors (pg. 118), and hip adductors (pg. 120). You should strengthen your quads and hip adductors only after your hamstrings and hip abductors are strong enough to offset the natural strength of these two muscle groups.

The knee is the joint most affected by a potential muscle imbalance, because the kneecap (patella) position is mostly determined by the length and tension of the quads (front thigh muscles). The patella glides through a groove as you bend and extend the knee. The amount of compression the patella develops in the joint depends on how much force the quads create on it and the length of the quads. A muscle-strength imbalance between the quads and hamstrings will affect both the compressive force and length of the quad.

If the quads are much stronger than the hamstrings—and they usually are—the quads will tend to shorten. As the quads shorten, the patella is pulled upward, creating greater compression between it and the *intercondylar groove* (the space the patella travels through at the end of the femur). As you bend your knee, the compressive force increases, causing the back of the patella to rub the joint. This creates excessive friction, which causes pain either behind or on the sides of the kneecap. You may feel a clicking sensation when you straighten or bend your knee, as the kneecap gets caught on the outside border of the groove it passes through. This is the number one issue I deal with when addressing knee pain. In most cases, when there's pain behind or around the kneecap, it's associated with the muscle imbalance between the quads and hamstrings; stretching the quads and strengthening the hamstrings resolves it fairly quickly.

Weaknesses in two other muscles also can cause knee pain—the *tensor fascia lata* and the *gastrocnemius*. The tensor fascia lata is a small hip abductor muscle that attaches at the top of the *iliotibial band* (ITB), a band of connective tissue that attaches to the side of the kneecap from the hip. This muscle is often weak in many people, and weakness can also cause a muscle to shorten. A strong muscle shortens because it has no opposing force to offset the excessive force, whereas a weak muscle has a tendency to become inflamed. Once inflamed, it thickens, losing its ability to maintain its proper length. The ITB attaches to the kneecap, drawing it laterally, pulling it more toward the outside edge of the groove it travels through, and increasing the friction between the lateral border of the groove and the kneecap.

This causes pain outside or beneath the kneecap. Strengthening the hamstrings and hip abductors helps resolve this pain.

The quads/hamstrings imbalance could also pull the kneecap deeper into its groove, causing pain. It's very rare for the hamstrings to be stronger than the quads, so strengthening the hamstrings along with the gastrocnemius, a calf muscle that passes the knee joint, should offset the imbalance and prevent the stronger quads from pulling on the kneecap. If you don't have pain at the kneecap, you can assume there's no muscle imbalance issue, and you can strengthen your quads as well. I prefer using squats or lunges (see Chapter 5) to achieve this goal, because they cause both the quads and hamstrings to contract. Activating both muscle groups simultaneously helps you maintain some form of balance, and it's a more stable way of strengthening the knee.

When strengthening the groin muscles to strengthen the knee, you need to consider the muscle balance between the hip abductors and adductors. Any muscle that's not balanced by its opposing muscle will have a tendency to shorten, and it won't be prepared to be stretch quickly enough. Because the adductors are often stronger than the abductors, excessively strengthening the adductors can lead to groin strains or tears. In all muscles there is a natural contractile force. In the case of two opposing muscles, the one with the greater contractile force will shorten. The weaker muscle will shorten only if it's inflamed. Most groin strains don't result from weak groin muscles; they result from weak hip abductors that can't offset the increased strength of the adductor. The adductors shorten excessively and are unable to stretch when you separate your legs.

It's unusual to experience pain at the joint between the femur and the *tibia* (lower leg bone) without some traumatic event triggering the pain. This joint is the site of the **meniscal cartilage**, the **anterior cruciate ligament** (ACL), and the posterior cruciate ligament (PCL). If you experience pain in this region, especially if it's the result of trauma, you should seek medical care.

Some structural deficits can also cause pain at the knee. They include arthritis, *chondromalacia patellae*, and a *meniscal tear*. Arthritis can form at any joint, especially if the surrounding muscles are weak. This makes the joint unstable, which causes the joint surfaces to rub together. This rubbing can irritate the joint surfaces, and eventually they wear down, marking the beginning of arthritis.

As with other joints, there are degrees of arthritis of the knee, and the arthritis is not necessarily what's causing the pain. If that were the cause, you'd lose both active and passive range of motion. You wouldn't be able to bend the knee as far as you would the other knee, and while you're relaxed, a second person wouldn't be able to move it. Arthritis of the knee typically affects the joint between the thighbone and lower leg bone. If you experience pain from arthritis, it would be along the inside or outside of the knee or on both sides. If your pain is around the kneecap or behind the kneecap, the pain is most likely not caused by arthritis.

Chondromalacia patellae is a softening of the cartilage on the back of the kneecap. All bones have a thin layer at the ends where they meet the joints. This smooth, hard substance, called *hyaline cartilage*, allows the surfaces of bones to bear force without deteriorating. If this cartilage softens, it can become inflamed and painful. Chondromalacia patellae is a common diagnosis when a patient complains of pain behind or on the side of the kneecap. But in my experience, there are two other common causes for knee pain: a muscle imbalance between the quads and hamstrings or an increased tightness of the ITB muscle. When a patient comes in with pain behind the kneecap, I perform a complete evaluation to determine whether the quads are much stronger and tighter than the hamstrings. If they are, I apply heat to the quads, massage it, then stretch it. Then, the patient frequently stands up and realizes the pain is substantially, if not completely, gone.

Torn meniscal cartilage is another overused diagnosis for knee pain, because the MRI is used as the overriding determining factor for the diagnosis. Regardless of the location of the pain, the manner of injury, or the clinical findings, if an MRI indicates a meniscal tear, the patient is told that surgery is required. I have several concerns with this scenario. First, MRIs are not perfect, nor are the individuals who read them. Second, the purpose of the MRI is to corroborate a clinical finding. In most of my cases, no clinical evaluation was performed. The patient was simply sent for an MRI, then a diagnosis was given. However, some tears are so minor that they don't require surgery.

Here's some information about the **meniscus** so you can better determine whether surgery is the appropriate course of action. The meniscus is a fibrous cartilage that sits between the thighbone and the lower leg bone. Its purpose is to act as a shock absorber to protect the knee from injury. The meniscus consists of two parts: one that sits to the outside of the knee (lateral) and one that sits to the inside (medial). The three most common ways of injuring your meniscus are by severely flexing (bending) your knee, by overextending (overstraightening) it, or by planting your foot on the floor and then excessively twisting it. The last one is common in skiing accidents or slipping on ice, where your foot is planted, and an external force causes your body to twist. If you can't determine that your symptoms were caused in this fashion, there's a good chance that you don't have a meniscal tear, or that if a tear was found on an MRI, it is not causing your pain and has probably been present for some time.

Symptoms of a meniscal tear are moderate to severe swelling at the knee joint and pain at the joint line on the side of the knee on which the meniscus was torn. You'd lose both active and passage range of motion from a meniscal tear. In most of my cases where the individual was misdiagnosed as having a meniscal tear, patients would complain of pain behind or around the kneecap. One individual had pain at the side of the knee, but it turned out to be a strained hamstring tendon. In most of these cases, the patients did not injure the meniscus.

Tearing a meniscus requires a trauma of reasonable severity. If that's the case, you should seek further assistance from a recommended orthopedic surgeon.

The Ankle

The muscle groups to strengthen to achieve and maintain a healthy ankle include the anterior tibialis (dorsiflexion and inversion) (pg. 129-130), calf muscles (plantarflexion) (pg. 126), posterior tibialis (inversion) (pg. 130), and peroneus muscles (eversion) (pg. 130).

Four main muscle groups help move and stabilize the ankle. The *dorsiflexors* and *plantar flexors* help create locomotion at the ankle and are responsible for the push-off portion of the walking cycle, when you're about to swing your leg forward to take the next step. The dorsiflexors bend the ankle up. When walking, this helps you to raise your toes and ankle as you swing your leg through to place your foot in front of your body and take the next step. The plantar flexors (calf muscles) bend the ankle down.

The other two muscle groups that stabilize the ankle are the *evertors* and *invertors*, which bend the ankle out and in, respectively. The invertors also help to support the arch of the foot to prevent flat-footedness.

The average person has no functional difficulties when it comes to the ankle, and most don't experience ankle pain unless they've experienced a traumatic event, such as a sprain, **shin splints**, a calf strain, **Achilles tendonitis**, or an ankle fracture.

The best way to maintain ankle function is to achieve a balance of strength with the opposing muscles: the dorsiflexors versus the plantar flexors and the invertors versus the evertors. In most cases, no additional strengthening is necessary. If your activities require excessive standing or walking, perform weight-training exercises to strengthen the four basic muscle groups of the ankle. These exercises help to support the joint and prevent any dysfunction or breakdown.

If you experience a sprain or fall, seek medical attention, because the pain associated with these types of traumas could be the result of a torn ligament or bone fracture. An x-ray or MRI is the proper course of action to determine whether structural damage has occurred and, if so, what the proper treatment protocol should be. The only other causes of pain associated with the ankle are from overuse syndromes or strains of the muscles surrounding the ankle. The muscle most often strained is the anterior tibialis, which can become inflamed and painful from excessive walking or running up inclines, or from simply running without proper conditioning. This is called shin splints because the inflamed muscle is just to the outside of the shinbone. Apply ice for a day or two to reduce the inflammation, and stay off your feet, then strengthen the anterior tibialis before resuming the activity.

In the case of calf cramps or strains, the problem is often not a weak calf muscle (gastrocnemius) but a weak anterior tibialis. This means that the calf muscles are stronger than their opposing muscle group, so the calf muscles shorten, losing their ability to create force and setting them up to strain or tear. This also sets up the Achilles tendon to be overstretched. Most cases of Achilles tendonitis I've treated occurred because the calf had become knotted and shortened due to a weak anterior tibialis. The increased pressure on the Achilles tendon causes it to become inflamed and painful.

You can also strain your calf muscles if you have a forward center of gravity due to muscle imbalances in both the upper and lower body. As your center of gravity moves in front of the ankle, you create an additional load for one or more muscles in the back of the body. When you weight bear through your ankle, your skeleton aligns to support your body weight. If you have a forward center of gravity, you weight bear more through the balls of your feet, and your skeleton doesn't pick up the additional load. Instead, your muscles—usually those of the calf—must work to support this load. If you're constantly straining your calf muscles or experiencing calf cramps, you could have a severely forward center of gravity. To correct this problem, you need to strengthen your glutes and hamstrings so the muscles of the back of the body pull your center of gravity back over the ankle. You also should strengthen your anterior tibialis, which sits just outside the tibia and crosses the ankle to extend down to the underside of the foot— to offset the tightness of the calf.

The Foot

The muscles to strengthen to resolve foot pain include the anterior and posterior tibialis (pg. 129-130), hip abductors (pg. 118), glutes (pg. 114, st. leg deadlifts), and hamstrings (pg. 112).

The most common foot pain is at the bottom of the foot, either just at the heel or from the heel to the ball of the foot. In most cases, it's the result of an inflamed **plantar fascia**, a band of connective tissue running from the heel to the ball of the foot. The plantar fascia helps to support the arch, the muscles within the foot, and the muscles that attach from the lower leg to the foot.

Most people with heel pain are diagnosed with a bone spur and told that the only treatment is a cortisone shot or an **orthotic** in the shoe. With almost every patient I've encountered, a bone spur wasn't the problem. Even if an x-ray showed a spur, the spur had been there for a while and wasn't responsible for the symptoms. What was causing the pain was an overstretched plantar fascia, which could result from weak anterior and posterior tibialis muscles or a severely forward center of gravity. As mentioned in the section on the ankle, a forward center of gravity causes you to weight bear more through the balls of your feet than your ankles.

Weak hip abductors also can cause the medial arch of the foot to flatten, overstretching the plantar fascia and causing heel pain. You're probably wondering how weakness at the hip region can cause foot pain. The answer is simple: the body is a chain of muscles working together to achieve proper weight bearing through all joints. If one area isn't functioning properly, that can cause another area to break down, creating pain. If your hip abductors are weak, then when you place one foot in front of another to take a step, your foot will move inside the line of the hip, and you'll be placing your weight more toward the outside of your foot. This forces the muscles on the inside of your foot—the anterior and posterior tibialis muscles—to work harder to bring your foot down as you weight bear on it. Over time, these muscles will break down, losing their ability to create force and support the arch of the foot. Once this occurs, the plantar fascia becomes overstretched and painful.

In some cases, weakness of the opposite-leg hip abductor can cause pain at the plantar fascia. This weakness causes the hip to drop, making you put more force through the foot than necessary. The anterior and posterior tibialis must support this increased force, and, once they can no longer handle the additional stress, you lose the arch of the foot and the plantar fascia becomes overstretched and painful.

Keep in mind that the body is a chain of joints working synergistically to create effective function. Your best chance of limiting pain and achieving full functional capacity is to keep all your joints healthy. To do this, you need to keep the surrounding musculature of all joints strong, flexible, and balanced with their opposing muscles. This will keep your joints in proper alignment, limiting possible irritation, and it will keep your muscles functioning efficiently. I have a large sign on the wall in my facility that says "Strength Equals Function." Learn it, live it, and experience a life free of pain.

4

THE GOLDEN RULES OF WEIGHT TRAINING

Before you even lift a barbell or a dumbbell, it's important to understand the basic guidelines for weight training. These are universal rules for all weight-training exercises. Follow them to achieve maximum benefit from each exercise and limit your chance of injury.

1. *Never lock a joint while weight training.* If you lock a joint (a position where's there's no bend at the joint), your skeletal system bears the weight load instead of your muscles. If you're bench-pressing, for instance, and you lock your elbow, the muscles no longer support the weight. The skeletal system takes over, and the weight gets transmitted from your hand through your arm bones and into your shoulder. When you release or unlock the elbow, pressure suddenly increases on the joint, because the bones aren't supporting the weight anymore; then the burden of the work is placed on both the **ligamentous tissue** (the ligaments or connective tissue that attach one bone to another at a joint)

and certainly the muscles. The sudden requirement for the muscles to contract and support the weight could result in a strain. Instead of building into a contraction in a continuous motion, the muscle has to contract instantly. If it can't, then the supporting soft tissue and ligaments must bear more of a load than usual. Only a couple of exercises, which we'll discuss later, require you to lock a joint to isolate a specific muscle. As a general rule, however, never lock a joint.

2. *Obtain a full range of motion when performing each exercise.* When performing an exercise, make sure the joint that the muscle moves goes through its full range of motion. If you're performing a biceps curl (see Chapter 5), for instance, start with your elbows slightly bent and bring the weight up until the dumbbell approaches your shoulder. Then return it to the starting position. The amount of work a muscle does depends not just on the weight it moves but also the distance it travels. So if you don't allow the joint that the muscle moves to go through its full range of motion, the muscle isn't performing its maximum work, and you're not allowing it to get stronger in the shortest period of time. Also, for every muscle there's an opposing muscle that moves the joint the opposite way. For the biceps, there are the triceps (the front and back of the arm), and for the quadriceps, there are the hamstrings (the front and back of the thigh). If you don't exercise the quadriceps through their full range of motion (for this muscle, that would be when your knee is fully straight but not locked), then the hamstrings aren't fully lengthened (see Figure 4.1). Over time, this can allow the hamstrings to shorten, setting the muscle up for a strain or a tear. As stressed earlier, do not use the amount of weight in these photos to determine the appropriate amount you should lift. These photos are to show proper form, not weight load.

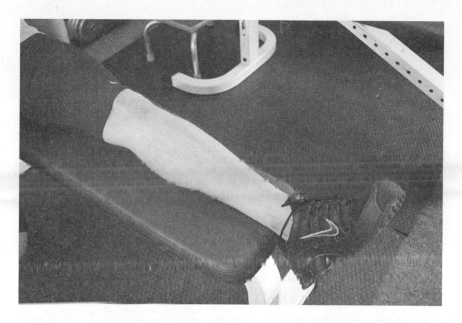

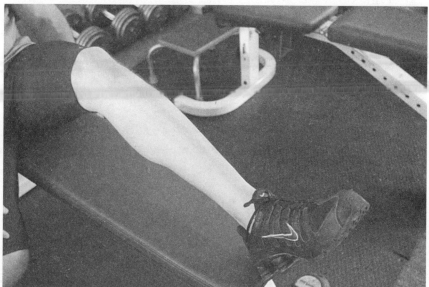

FIGURE 4.1 (a) First photo indicates a knee joint with full range of muscle resulting from strengthening the quadriceps through full range of motion. (b) Second photo indicates hamstrings that are shortened due to not working the quadriceps through full range of motion.

3. *Achieve a controlled, slow motion when performing an exercise.*
   If you build up momentum during an exercise, the momentum will provide the motion and work, not the muscle. Therefore, your muscle will be less efficient at gaining strength. Another reason not to build momentum is to avoid sending your brain the wrong signals. Muscles contract as a result of nerve receptors in a joint. These receptors let the brain know how much stress there is on the joint as a result of lifting the weight. The brain then sends a signal to the muscle to contract, stabilize, and move the joint. If you build momentum, you limit the amount of signaling that goes from the joint receptors to the brain. This limits the brain's understanding of how much stress you've placed on the joint and limits the amount of nerve impulse transmission to the muscle. The lower the amount of nerve impulse transmission to the muscle, the less it can contract and get stronger. To avoid building momentum, concentrate on involving only the muscle you're working in the lift; don't jerk the weight at the beginning of the lift and maintain a consistent speed throughout the set.

4. *Use the appropriate amount of weight.* The best way to describe this rule is if you don't feel like you're doing anything, you're probably not. If you're using a certain resistance and you don't feel like you've done any work by the end of your set, you should increase the weight. If your target is twelve to fifteen repetitions and you can perform twenty, thirty, or forty with that weight, increase the weight. Another way of knowing that you're not using enough weight is if you can talk to someone through the whole set. If the weight is appropriate, you'll have to concentrate on your lift to avoid injury. Conversely, if you can't control the weight, you're using too much. If you can't hit the target number of repetitions you're shooting for in a set, the weight is too great. Choosing the right weight lets

you perform the right number of repetitions in each set to get the most out of each set.

5. *Don't perform more than two or three exercises for each body part.* There's a misconception that more is better when weight training. Each muscle performs a very specific function. It moves in a simple pattern. It doesn't take more than two or three exercises to maximally work each muscle. Weight training is all about intensity. If you perform only one exercise for each muscle group, as long as you're using sufficient weight and increasing the weight after each set, you're going to grow muscle. One exercise for a body part should be considered a minimum requirement. Some experts say you have to work each muscle from different angles to work all the fiber in a muscle. This is simply untrue. The fibers pull together to form one line of pull on the muscle. If you make the muscle pull along this line, you'll get all the muscle fiber to pull in a maximum effort without going to different angles and wasting time and energy.

    Performing an exercise with dumbbells and then barbells is also inefficient. Dumbbells are separate weights for each hand, while a barbell has a weight attached at each end. I prefer dumbbells, because they require more stability. The extra work required to stabilize the dumbbells produces more nerve impulses. Because it's the nerve impulses that cause a muscle to contract, dumbbells offer the best opportunity to use all of a muscle's fiber to move the weight. What's more, dumbbells allow joints to go through a normal range of motion, whereas a barbell can inhibit the motion of a joint by tying the two hands together.

6. *Perform every exercise on a single plane.* Each muscle performs one or two primary functions. The biceps flexes the elbow (by bending your elbow, you bring your hand to your shoulder) and, to a lesser extent, turns your palm upward or "supinates"

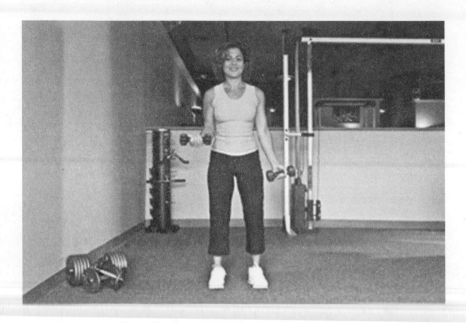

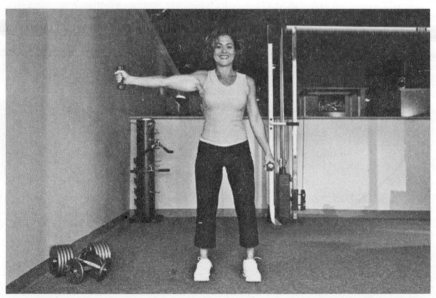

FIGURE 4.2 (a) First photo shows exercise being performed in the frontal plane. (b) Second photo shows exercise being performed in the sagittal plane.

your hand. The deltoid raises your arm out from your side and up over your head. Each of these motions occurs on a single plane. The biceps works on a plane that goes from the front of the body to the back (the frontal plane); the deltoid goes from side to side (the sagittal plane) (see Figure 4.2).

I see people in the gym rotating their forearms as they raise their arms. They're losing a tremendous amount of energy performing that rotational movement, and they're not getting any value out of it. Basically, you should perform a motion on a single plane, and no other movements, such as rotation, should occur. A good rule of thumb is if a movement feels difficult because it's too complex, then something's wrong. Every exercise being performed when weight training should be very simple. The movements are very basic. If you work on a plane from the front of your body to the back, as in a biceps curl, for example, you should see no motion from side to side or on a rotational or transverse plane.

7. *Lift so your force directly opposes the weight.* Always lift so the force you create directly opposes the weight you're trying to lift. When bench-pressing (see Chapter 5), for instance, people ask whether they should use a narrow or a wide grip when they hold the bar. The answer is neither. You should place your hands on the bar so you can directly oppose the resistance you're pushing against; in this case, the weight is pushing directly down. You should place your hands so your forearms are directly perpendicular to the floor. This allows you to push directly opposite the weight. Any other position redirects some of your force out to the side or in toward you. In either case, you won't be able to lift your maximum resistance. Another example is a lat pulldown (see Chapter 5). People think positioning their hands further out on the bar is better. This is incorrect. Place your hands on the bar so your forearms are perpendicular to the floor. This way, you're pulling directly

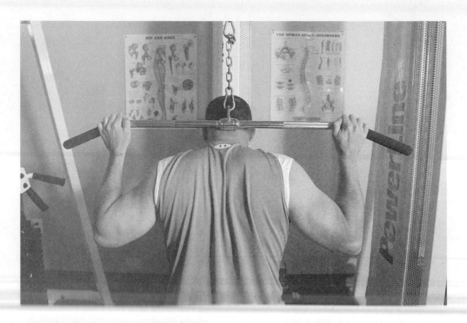

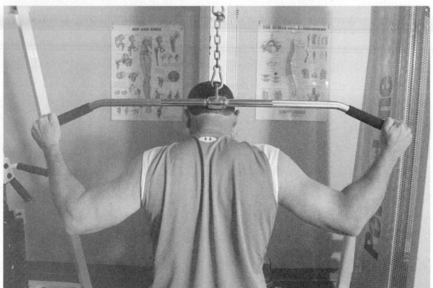

FIGURE 4.3 (a) The photo on the top shows the right way to hold the bar when doing a lat pulldown. (b) The photo at the bottom shows the wrong way.

opposite the resistance, which, in this case, is pulling directly upward (see Figure 4.3).

8. *Make sure you're in a stable and safe position when exercising.* When you perform any exercise, only one side of the muscle should be moving; the other side should be stable. Therefore, a large portion of your body should be stable, and only the joints involved in the exercise should be moving. The best position for doing biceps curls, for instance, is seated, because every part of your body other than the elbow you're flexing has the opportunity to be flat, stable, and not moving. When you're in proper position, there's less chance of incorporating other muscle groups. When you're well-balanced and stable, you can concentrate your energy on lifting the resistance, not balancing and supporting the rest of your body. Take bench-pressing. You can lift more when your feet are flat on the floor than when they're up on the bench, because your base of support is much greater. Because your body is more stable, you can devote more energy to the actual lift. When your feet are up, you're expending energy trying to keep yourself from falling off the bench. This is energy you could be using to lift for maximum efficiency.

9. *If you're working more than one body part a day, always work the larger body part first.* This is especially true if you're trying to increase your mass. Because you'll incorporate more resistance when performing the exercise for the larger body part, you'll require more energy. If you work the smaller body part first, you may not have enough energy left for the larger body part, and you won't have an efficient workout. Your own efficiency and energy levels will dictate the optimal number of body parts you should exercise in a day. I've found it's almost impossible for me to do more than two body parts in a day. I also try to get out of the gym in ninety minutes. I'm not able to sustain a high level of energy for more than ninety minutes.

If I go beyond two hours, I'm too tired and can't achieve my maximum efficiency in the exercise. I'm comfortable getting my two body parts done during a ninety-minute period. Some people have the opportunity to do only one body part at a time. It's a matter of time constraints and your lifestyle. I have a pretty hectic schedule, and I've found this to be the best workout routine for me. It's important to create a schedule you can stick with that also suits your needs.

10. *Allow a muscle enough time to rest and grow before working it again.* The rehabilitation of muscle doesn't occur while you're performing an exercise; it comes after that. The healing and rebuilding of muscle fiber begins the day after you perform the exercise. If you train the same muscle during this process, you could limit the muscle's ability to develop more muscle tissue and make the muscle more susceptible to injury. I've reduced the number of workouts I perform in a week from six days to five and now to four. If you work each body part once a week, that's enough to cause growth. I hit every upper body part every five days. The soreness lasts for two days, and, by the fifth day, I've allowed for a total recovery, and the muscle is ready to be worked again. I don't believe in the concept of doing a light day and a heavy day of weight. If you've rested properly, there's no need for that, and there's no chance of causing injury. I work my legs only once a week, because I work them to such an extreme level that it usually takes two to three days for them to recover. For the same reasons, I don't believe you should work any body part more than twice a week. Anything more than that will not allow a sufficient amount of recovery time. You're inviting a breakdown or injury.

11. *Always keep the weight close to the part of your body through which you're transmitting resistance to the floor.* When performing exercises where you're running the weight along your body, such as straight-leg dead lifts, **posterior deltoids**, and barbell

rows (see Chapter 5), keep the weight close to your body. If you bring the weight any distance in front or behind your legs, for instance, you're no longer transmitting the weight directly through your legs (see Figure 4.4).

Something instead of your legs has to work to support the weight, and inevitably, it's your lower back. If you're doing a barbell row—an exercise where you bend forward and lift a weight along your legs to your stomach—and if you keep the weight in front of you and away from your legs, your lower back muscles will have to support the weight in an awkward position, which could cause an injury.

Try this yourself: Take a very small weight, bend forward, and place the weight right in front of your legs. Now slowly move the weight in front of you away from your legs. As the weight gets farther and farther from you, you can feel your lower back muscles working to support it. To avoid potential injury and lift the maximum amount of weight, you need to avoid involving your lower back in the lift. You can also see this in the squat, an exercise where you hold the weight on your shoulders and squat down until your thighs are parallel to the floor. Here, you're transmitting resistance to the floor through your heels. If the weight gets in front of your ankles, you'll feel yourself getting pulled forward onto your toes. The only muscles that can stop this from happening are those of your lower back. Again, this is inefficient and can cause injury.

12. *If you feel pain while stretching, you're stretching too hard.* Pain while stretching is an indication that you're performing with too much tension, and the muscle is contracting to limit the pain. You can't achieve a high level of stretch when the muscle is contracting. A stretch should be a very comfortable sensation. The effect should be mild, and you should be able to sustain it. The old saying "no pain, no gain" doesn't apply here.

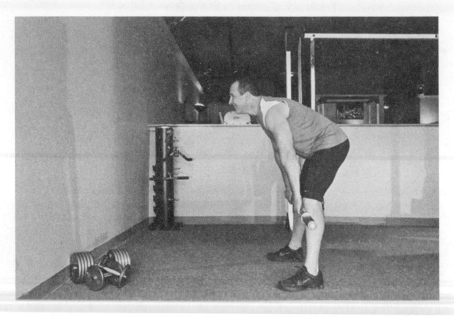

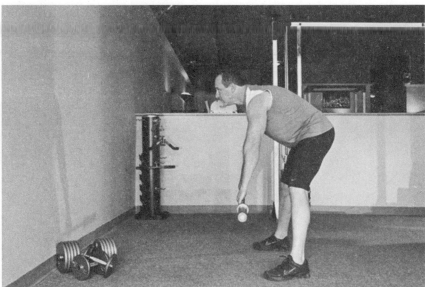

Figure 4.4 (a) First photo shows resistance being kept close to the body. (b) Second photo shows resistance being maintained away from the body, creating an additional load for the lower back to support.

13. *When stretching or strengthening your legs, keep the knee of your front leg in line with your foot, never in front of it.* When squatting, doing lunges, doing a quad stretch or other exercise incorporating the leg, your knee should not pass in front of your foot. If it does, you could injure your knee. In terms of strengthening, you won't achieve the maximum efficiency of the quadriceps unless your knee stays as close to over your heel as possible. In addition, your shin should remain as close to perpendicular to the floor as possible. This gives the quadriceps their greatest mechanical advantage to create force (see Figure 4.5).

14. When performing an exercise, always set the speed of the eccentric portion of a motion at one and a half times slower than the concentric portion of the motion. When a muscle lengthens, that's called the eccentric portion of a movement. When it shortens, that's the concentric portion. When performing a biceps curl, for instance, raising your hand up toward your shoulder is the concentric portion of the exercise, and lowering your hand back down is the eccentric portion. The eccentric portion should take one and a half times longer than the concentric phase of the movement, because most injuries occur during the lengthening phase and more care is necessary at this time.

15. Always exhale during the portion of the exercise where the muscle is shortening. For instance, forcibly exhale as you bring the weight up toward the shoulder when performing a biceps curl and as you raise the weights overhead when performing a military press (see Chapter 5). The shortening phase of a muscle typically occurs when working against gravity if using free weights. The purpose of the forced exhale is twofold. First, if you hold your breath while lifting weights, arterial and venous pressure can increase in the brain and potentially cause injury. Second, a forced exhale causes your abdominal muscles

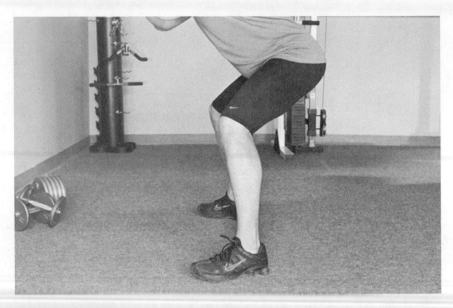

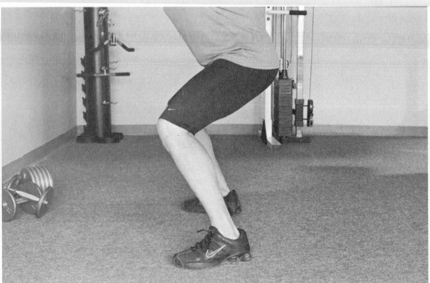

FIGURE 4.5 (a) Maintain the knee over, (b) not in front of, the ankle while performing squats, lunges, and quads stretches.

to contract hard, making this region more stable. A stable torso and pelvis enhances your ability to lift weights with your arms or legs. This is because your thigh muscles ultimately attach to your pelvis, and your arm muscles ultimately attach to your shoulders, which are the end points of your torso. As you use your muscles to move weights, an opposing force will try to move your torso or pelvis toward the weights you're lifting. The stabilizing muscles of your torso and pelvis can offset this force. The muscles that can be most critically affected by using a breathing technique are the abdominal muscles. The only exceptions to this rule are exercises for the shoulders— shrugs and front, side, and posterior laterals. In these cases, you should inhale when the muscles are shortening.

5

ENOUGH TALK—LET'S GET TO WORK!

The exercises in this chapter cover the main muscle groups—chest, back, biceps, legs, shoulders, and triceps—as well as the minor ones—abdominals, forearms, and calves. For each muscle group, I'll discuss the attachments of the muscles and their function, and I'll explain the exercises you should perform to strengthen the muscles of that group. Don't worry if you don't have a gym membership. A small investment in a set of dumbbells, a bench, and a pair of ankle cuff weights will enable you to perform most of these exercises. And don't worry about a workout schedule yet; we'll cover that in Chapter 7.

The Chest

The main muscle of the chest is the pectoralis major—known as the pecs. This fan-shaped muscle attaches to the sternum (breastbone), clavicle (collarbone), and several ribs at one end and to the medial border of the bicipital groove on the humerus (the inside of the upper arm bone) at the other. Simply put, it attaches from the torso to the arm. The main function of the pecs is horizontal adduction. (Adduction occurs when you bring your arms toward the midline of your torso; abduction when bring your arms away from the midline of your body.) The best way to describe this motion is that of a bear hug. To give the most effective bear hug—to use the pecs most efficiently—your elbows should be level with your shoulders. The shoulder's normal range of motion of horizontal abduction is 100 degrees. We'll reinforce this when I describe the individual exercises.

The three most important exercises for strengthening the pecs are the flat bench or bench press, the flat-bench flye, and the incline bench press. If time is tight, you can eliminate the incline bench press. That exercise is more for the serious weight trainer who's looking to shape the pecs, and you can achieve good results with just the flat bench and flye.

Bench Press: The most popular exercise for strengthening the chest is the flat bench, also called the bench press. To do it right, you need to position your shoulders, elbows, and hands properly. Let's start with the hand position. Remember, to create the greatest amount of force against the resistance, you need to push directly opposite the resistance. In this case, that is with your forearms perpendicular to the ground. You might have been told to use a wide grip or a narrow grip or even of varying your grips. Forget all that. As for your elbows, they should be in line with your shoulders. If they start to come down toward your sides, you end up using more front delt and triceps than you do pecs. So to isolate the pecs, keep those elbows in line with your shoulders. The common belief has been that, as you bring the bar down toward your chest, you bring the bar across the nipple line. But that encourages you to bring your elbows toward your sides, which prevents you from isolating or maximizing the use of the pecs. Don't concern

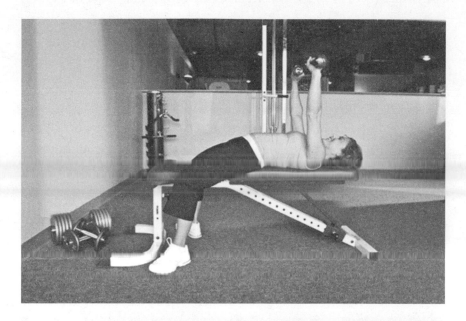

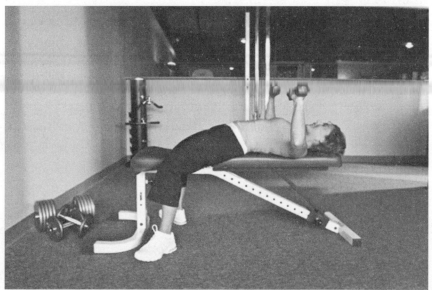

FIGURE 5.1 Bench press. The start, above, and the finish, below.

yourself with where the bar comes down. As long as your elbows are in line with your shoulders, let the bar come down to wherever is comfortable. When you're pushing up, don't push straight up. The weight should actually go up and slightly backward. Because of the anatomy of the shoulder, this is the most natural arc created when performing this exercise.

With your elbows facing out and your forearms perpendicular to the ground, lower the weight down to your chest, concentrating on keeping your elbows in line with your shoulders. Don't focus too much on controlling the weight down, but don't allow it to just fall either. Bring the weight up to the top position, which is just before you lock your elbows. Don't push the weight back up too quickly, because a fast motion relies more on momentum than muscle.

Flat-Bench Flye: Another popular chest exercise is the flye movement. Make sure your hands never extend past your elbows as you lower the weight, because this places a tremendous amount of rotational force or *torque* on your shoulders as the weight is increased by the length of the arm. This torque causes stress on the front of the shoulder joint. Most people think this sensation is the pecs being worked. Actually, it's more the anterior shoulder or capsule being stretched, which prevents you from pushing as much resistance and maximizing the use of the pecs.

Another misconception about the flye movement is that you have to bring your hands way out to get a maximum stretch of the pecs. But when you understand that the pecs attach from the torso to the upper arm, you realize that as long as the elbow goes as far back as it can, you'll get the proper stretch. Your hand position doesn't come into play.

With the weights overhead and your palms facing inward, slowly control the weights out. Your elbows will bend, your hands will stay over your elbows, and your elbows will come out in line with

73

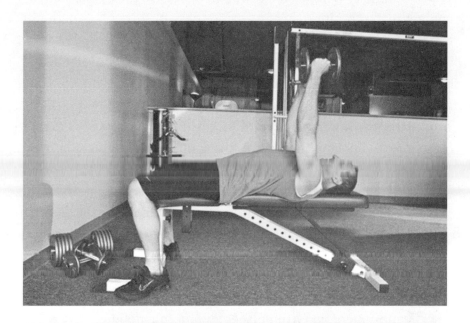

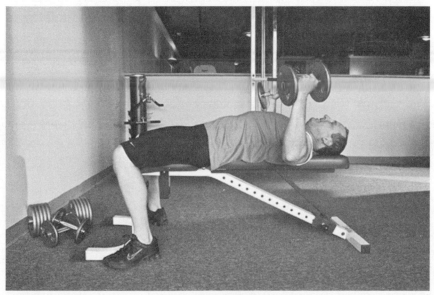

FIGURE 5.2 Flye. The start, above, and the finish, below.

your shoulders. When you feel a stretch, begin to bring the weights up to the start position, just before your elbows lock. There should be no rotational movement in the course of this exercise. As long as you're creating a horizontal adduction motion, you'll be using the pecs in their most efficient manner.

Incline Press: If you really want to maximize the development of your chest, you can also perform the incline press. There's a separation between the upper and lower pecs, and this exercise enables you to isolate the upper pecs. Many people, myself included, find that their lower pecs are naturally more developed and that the upper pecs need additional strengthening to even out the shape of the chest. (While sitting on a bench with the back on an incline works the upper pecs, sitting at a 90-degree angle works the deltoids—more on that later.)

The movement and hand placement for the incline press are basically the same as for the bench press. The most comfortable angle at which to perform the exercise, however, varies by individual. For most, 30 degrees is a comfortable angle. As with the flat bench, you want to keep your forearms perpendicular to the floor and your elbows in line with your shoulders, and again control the weight both up and down in a proper rhythm. As with the flat bench, the weight should go up and slightly backward as you push up.

The Abdominal Group

People use all types of equipment to work their abdominal muscles, but the mistake I see most often is the movement that is occurring from the hip. To understand how to isolate the abdominal muscles, it helps to know where each muscle is and what it does.

The *rectus abdominis* attaches from the underside of the ribs, as well as the sternum, iliac, and pubic region of the pelvis (see Figure 5.4).

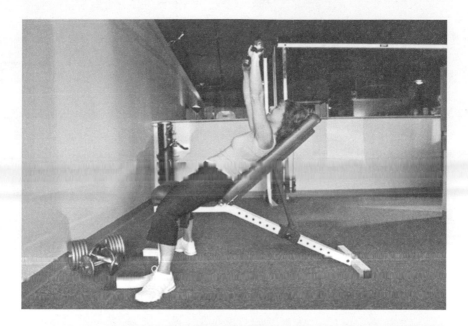

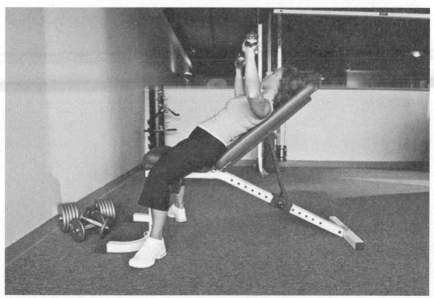

FIGURE 5.3 Incline press. The start, above, and the finish, below.

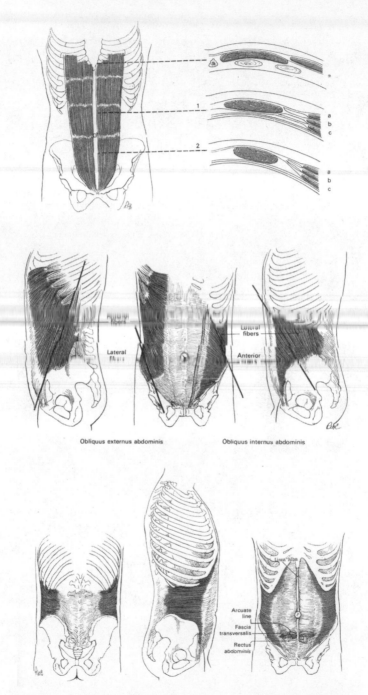

Obliquus externus abdominis   Obliquus internus abdominis

FIGURE 5.4 (a), (b), (c) Photos of abdominal muscles and connections.

The abdominal wall is an intertwining of the rectus abdominis and several other muscles, including the *obliques.* These other muscles contract as stabilizers when you do the modified sit-up—or trunk curl—I'm about to describe. That means the rectus abdominis contracts to perform the movement, and the other muscles contract to keep the pelvis and ribs moving in proper alignment.

The most frequent question I get about working the abdominals is: How often can I work them? The answer is simple. Like any muscle other than the heart, the abdominals are skeletal muscles. So you should work them just as often as you would any other skeletal muscles—twice a week. If you really want to be aggressive, three times a week is the maximum.

Another oft asked question is: How many repetitions should I do in a set? Again, go back to your other muscles. You don't do two hundred or three hundred bench presses or biceps curls in a set. So why do that many sit-ups? Limit the reps to ten per set and no more.

You should also progress in weight just as you would with the other muscles, by increasing the resistance as the muscles get stronger. The resistance comes from the weights you cradle on your chest with your arms. Increase the weights as you adapt to them.

Modified Sit-up (Trunk Curl): The modified sit-up and reverse trunk curl are all you need to build the abdominal region. The modified situp exercise works both the upper and lower abdominal muscles. Lie on your back with your knees bent. Put your hands either behind your neck or across your chest. You utilize resistance by clutching a weight at your chest. As you advance, you can clutch increasing amounts of weight. Lift your head, neck, and shoulders up until the lowest point of your shoulder blade is off the floor. Keep your lower back on the floor at all times to protect it from stress; you're just curling the top portion of your trunk up. To create this movement, your abdominals muscles have

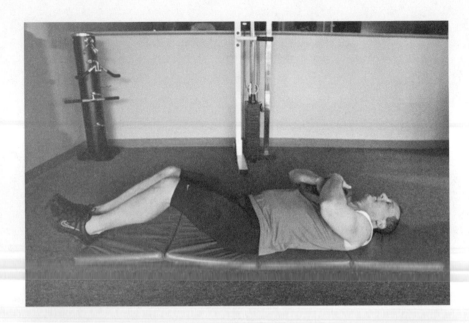

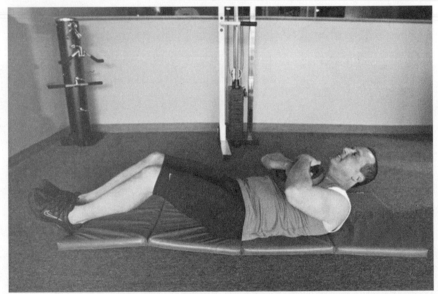

FIGURE 5.5 Trunk curl. The start, above, and the finish, below.

to contract. To stabilize the pelvis during the exercise, point your toes up so only your heel remains on the floor and dig your heel into the floor to help reinforce it. This forces your glutes (butt muscles) to contract, locking your pelvis in place and allowing the rectus abdominis to pull from the pelvis to raise the torso. While your torso is curling up, notice that the angle between your pelvis and your torso does not change. This eliminates the chance of compensating for weak abdominals by using the hip flexors to perform the exercise.

You can perform this exercise on a flat bench or on the floor. Regardless of which you choose, the key is to not move from the hip. The trunk curl is a very small motion that surprises most people. At the height of the movement, your head should be no more than 60 degrees above your pelvis (see Figure 5.6).

One of the biggest complaints I get from people trying to perform the trunk curl is that they feel stress in their necks. This is because they're hyperflexing the neck by tucking the chin into the chest. To avoid overstretching the back of the neck, pretend there's a tennis ball between your chin and chest. This will keep your neck in its proper position.

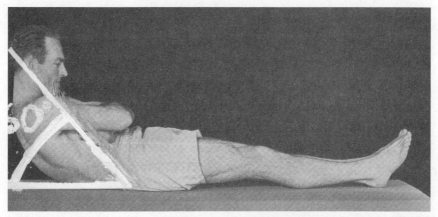

FIGURE 5.6 When performing a trunk curl, the angle between your head and torso should be no more than 60 degrees.

Reverse Trunk Curl: This exercise lets you isolate the lower portion of your abdominal muscles. If you're performing the exercise on the floor, place your hands at your sides. If you're doing the movement on a bench, hold onto the foot support or end of the bench behind your head. With your legs perpendicular to the floor and your feet flexed (toward your face), try to raise your heels toward the ceiling. What you're doing is actually the reverse of a trunk curl. Although extremely small, this movement is very difficult to master. The lower abdominal region is very thin and therefore has little ability to create force. If worked properly, this could help pull in that little bulge at the bottom of your abdominal region just below your belly button. You raise the resistance by using ankle weights, increasing the weight as you progress.

Trunk Curl with Rotation: An additional exercise you can perform is the trunk curl with rotation. This will isolate the obliques—a small muscle group at the sides of the abdominal region. You perform this exercise the same way you do the trunk curl, from a lying-down position. The only difference is that you keep one shoulder on the floor or bench while raising the other one toward the opposite knee. Lift one shoulder completely off the floor or bench while keeping the other one on the floor or bench throughout the exercise. You can do one side at a time or alternate sides. You increase resistance the same way you would with the trunk curl. Repetitions are also the same as for the trunk curl.

The machines you see in the gym and advertised on television will never be as effective as the trunk curl. Even leg raises can't cause the abdominal muscles to act as the primary mover the way the trunk curl does. To strengthen the abdominal region, you must do trunk curls, reverse trunk curls, and—if you are ambitious enough—trunk curls with rotation. Those torso-twisting machines that you hold onto and rotate don't work the obliques as described. You must have trunk flexion and rotation together to work the obliques.

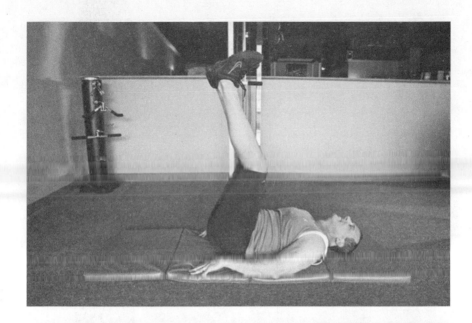

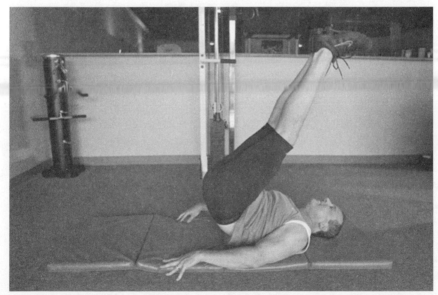

FIGURE 5.7 Reverse trunk curl. The start, above, and the finish, below.

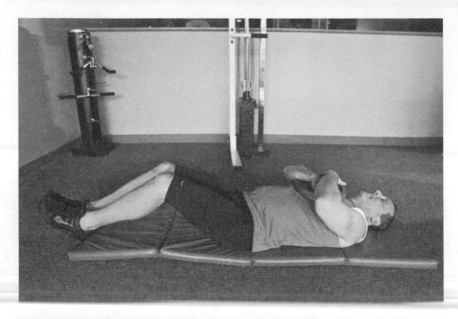

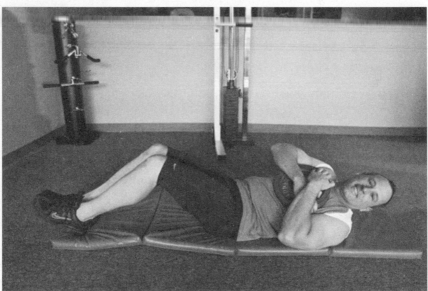

FIGURE 5.8 Trunk curl with rotation. The start, above, and the finish, below.

The Back

The back muscles are made up of three major groups. The upper back consists of the *posterior deltoids*, *rhomboids*, and *middle trapezius* (mid-trap) area. The *latissimus dorsi* (lats) and *teres major* make up the mid back. And the *erector spinae* and *quadratus lumborum* make up the lower back.

The largest of the three muscle groups of the back is the mid back. The teres major attaches from the side of the shoulder blade to the upper arm. The lats attach from several of the vertebrae and a fascia (a thick connective tissue in the lower back) to the upper portion of the pelvis. All of these areas join and connect to the upper arm (see Figure 5.9).

The functions of the lats and teres major are adduction and extension of the shoulder. During adduction, you bring your arms from straight out at your sides and parallel to the floor, down to your sides. During extension, you bring your arms from a position straight out in front of you and parallel to the floor, down toward your body. The shoulder has 180 degrees of adduction and 210 degrees of extension.

People use all kinds of equipment and all manner of grips to strengthen the mid back, but you need only two basic exercises to properly work the lats and teres major: one incorporating shoulder extension and another incorporating shoulder adduction.

Behind-the-Neck Pulldown: This exercise is an adduction of the teres major and lats. The pecs are also involved in this movement, but because the mechanical position is not as good for the pecs as it is for the lats and teres major, it's not considered a pecs exercise.

Start by grabbing the bar so your forearms will be perpendicular to the floor while going through the range of motion. Again, you want to pull directly opposite the pull of the resistance. In this

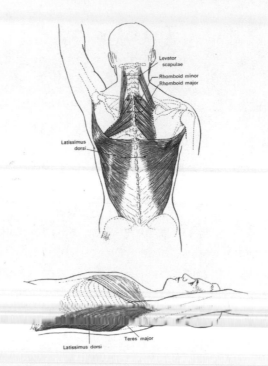

FIGURE 5.9 Illustration of latissimus dorsi/teres major and attachments.

case, the resistance is trying to pull upward, so you want to be in the best position to pull downward. One of the most common misconceptions is that you're supposed to grab the bar as widely as possible to get the maximum growth of your lats. In fact, you simply have to make them pull the greatest amount of resistance possible. By now, you know this means pulling directly opposite the pull of the resistance.

To ensure the greatest amount of stability, set the cushion so it's snug against your thighs. Lean slightly forward so you can bring the bar down behind your head to your neck. You're in the right position if the cable attached to the bar comes straight down. As you lower the bar toward your neck, make sure your elbows come down to an imaginary point at the sides of your body, not behind the line of your shoulders. This is where many people make a mis-

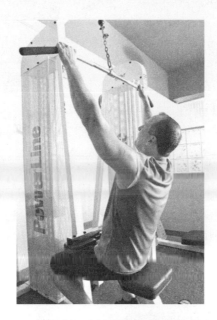

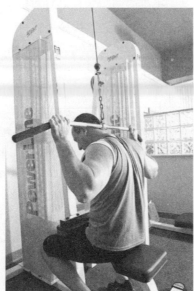

FIGURE 5.10 Behind-the-neck pulldown. The start, above, and the finish, below.

take. If your elbows get behind your shoulders, you'll be drawing the head of the humerus forward and you'll feel tightness at the front of your shoulder. The result can be stretched ligaments at the front of the shoulders, as well as tendonitis resulting from compressed tendons. You'll also begin to incorporate muscles you're not trying to work—those between your shoulder blades. By working these muscles, you're not fully working the lats and the teres major.

As the weight comes up to the start point, let your shoulders come up slightly. By allowing the shoulders to elevate, you maximize the stretch on the lats and teres major and enable better strengthening of the two muscles.

Seated Pulley Row: There's a lot of confusion as to what should occur at the torso as you perform this exercise. I see people bringing their chest all the way forward almost to the point where they're touching their knees and also bringing their back all the way to where they're lying backward. Because the lats and teres major don't pass the hip joint, putting this joint through a full range of motion doesn't strengthen these muscles. All the torso attachments are somewhere above the hips—whether the attachment is at the vertebrae, the **thoracolumbar fascia**, or the **iliac crest**.

To perform this exercise properly, grab the bar in both hands. Lean slightly back so your shoulders are positioned behind your hips when looking at them from the side. Keep your knees slightly bent. Start with your arms almost fully extended in front of you, with your elbows just unlocked. Begin to pull the bar back to your stomach, keeping your elbows running along the sides of your body until they've passed beyond your back. Then, slowly control the bar back to its start position, with your arms in front of you and your elbows unlocked.

The hip area should remain stable. The primary movers should be the arms, which is where the lats and teres major attach. Keep

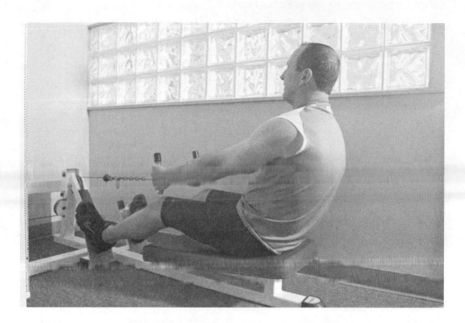

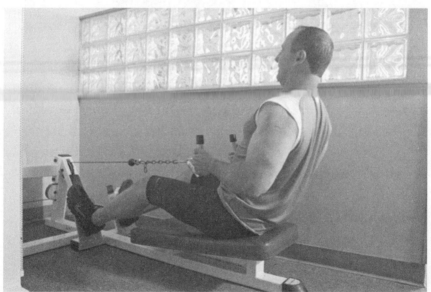

FIGURE 5.11 Seated pulley row. The start, above, and the finish, below.

your arms moving in a motion of extension and bring your elbows toward the back of your body, almost touching your body. All the motion should occur from the arms; the torso should not move forward or back. Once you're in the seated position, the angle of your torso should never change (see Figure 5.12).

The only thing that should change with regard to the torso is that you should go from a hunched position at the start of the exercise to an arched position at the finish. To maximize the stretch and get the best range of motion for the lats and teres major, bring your arms out to initiate the motion and hunch your back slightly. You'll round out your back, but your hip position won't change.

Your shoulder should protract by bringing your arm bone forward in the shoulder joint. Again, this will elongate the lats and teres for the greatest range of motion. As you bring your elbows back, you'll begin to retract your shoulders slightly and arch your back. As you do this, you're shortening the muscles. To complete the motion, your elbows should end up either directly in line with your back or slightly behind it. As you go behind your back, you'll start to feel your shoulder blades come together. You'll actually be getting more of the rhomboids/mid-traps involved in this motion. This is okay, and in fact, beneficial, because you're incorporating these additional muscle groups after the lats and teres major have completed their work.

Upper Back

The muscles of the upper back—the posterior deltoids, rhomboids, and mid-traps—perform horizontal abduction. You achieve this by bringing your arms behind you just below shoulder height. Weak upper back muscles cause your shoulders to come forward. By strengthening these muscles, you're keeping your shoulders back for better posture. These muscles also support your head, and weakness in these muscles can cause headaches. Whether you use

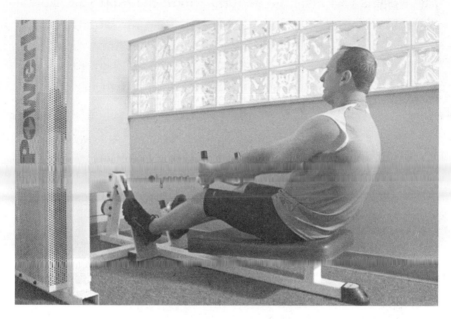

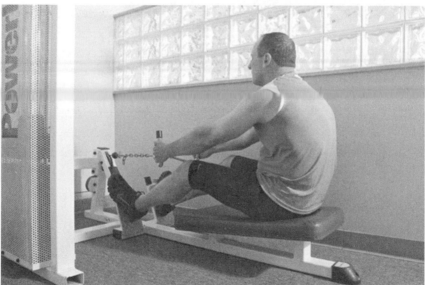

FIGURE 5.12 (a) The picture on the top shows the correctly maintained torso position. (b) The picture on the bottom shows the torso moving forward incorrectly.

free weights or a machine, if you perform the proper horizontal abduction, you can't go wrong. My favorite is the lat pulldown in front with a neutral bar.

Lat Pulldown in Front with Neutral Bar: You can perform this exercise with the regular lat pulldown bar, but I prefer a neutral bar (see Figure 5.14), because you can hold your elbows outward in a better position to complete the exercise. Grab the regular lat pulldown bar wider than you would for the behind-the-neck

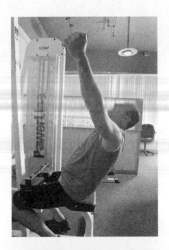

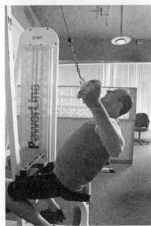

FIGURE 5.13 Lat pulldown in front with neutral bar.

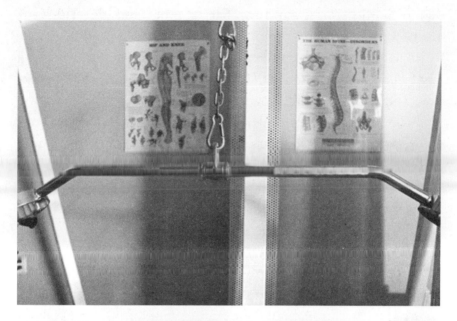

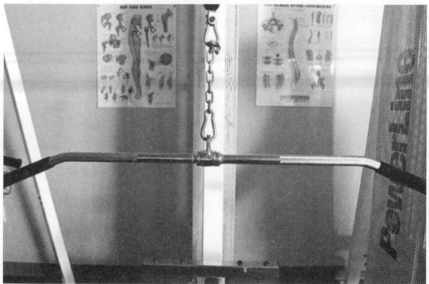

FIGURE 5.14 (a) Neutral bar and (b) lat pulldown bar.

pulldown. If using the neutral bar, grab the handle inside the U-shaped portion of the bar. Lean back slightly, and start with your back slightly hunched.

Begin to bring the bar toward your chin, keeping your elbows just below shoulder height. This will create a motion that causes your shoulder blades to squeeze together. If your elbows are too low, you won't feel this sensation. As you pull the bar toward your chin, arch your back to get the maximum range of motion. There are only about 20 degrees of motion once you get behind the line of the shoulders, so you won't be bringing your elbows very far behind you. Bring the bar toward your chin until you feel your shoulder blades squeeze together. It's okay if you don't reach your chin when this occurs; you've achieved the goal of the exercise when you get your shoulders to come together. Slowly return the bar to the start position while slowly going from arching to hunching your back. Throughout the exercise, your torso should remain in the same position, you shouldn't be swaying forward or back to assist in moving the bar. If you are, you're using too much weight.

Lower Back

Most people believe it's essential to strengthen the lower back. I disagree. By using your lower back to lift, you risk injury. What's more, if you overstrengthen these muscles, they can overcome their opposing muscle group, the abdominal muscles. This can reinforce an increased arch of the lower back, which causes the lower back muscles to shorten, making them ineffective and susceptible to muscle strain. It also causes poor posture, which can lead to injuries.

The lower back has two functions: to transmit weight from the upper body to the lower body to the floor and to stabilize the torso and allow the arms or legs to push off a stable surface. Any time

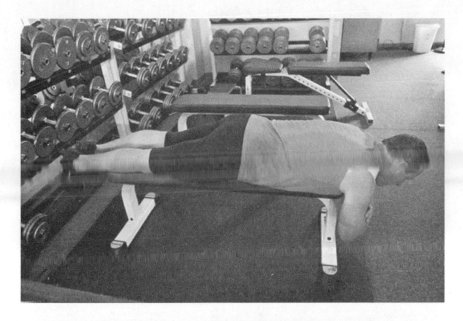

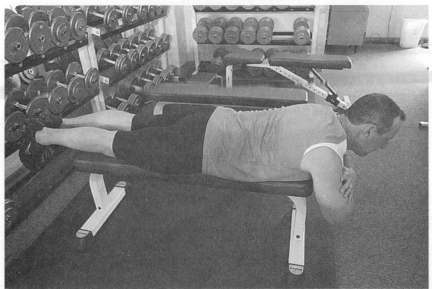

FIGURE 5.15 Hyperextensions. The start, above, and the finish, below.

you perform an exercise that works your arms or legs, your lower back muscles are activated to work as stabilizing muscles.

One more point about the lower back muscles: because of the way the joints of the torso and hip are positioned, the lower back muscles must constantly contract to keep your torso from falling forward when sitting or standing. So you're strengthening these muscles through constant use. If you decide to strengthen your lower back muscles through exercise, I strongly recommend that you equally strengthen your abdominal muscles.

Hyperextensions: The best way to perform this exercise is lying on your stomach. With your arms at your sides, raise your head and chest off the floor until you feel an arch in your lower back and then return to the floor. The lower back muscles simply arch the torso, and there are only about 60 degrees of movement. Anything more must occur from the hip. If you perform this exercise incorrectly, your glutes and hamstrings are doing the work and your lower back is simply stabilizing the torso to allow you to lift it.

Entire Back

No back workout is complete without some type of rowing exercise: either the barbell row, the T-bar row, or the one-arm row. These really are the main mass builders, incorporating all the muscles of the back.

Barbell Row: This is probably the most difficult of the three. Standing with knees slightly bent and butt back so you're in a semi-seated position, grip a barbell so your forearms can pull directly perpendicular to the floor. This ensures that you use the full strength of the lats and teres major. Feet should be a little more than shoulder width apart, and you should feel yourself weight bearing mostly on your heels. Bend forward at the waist just enough so your shoulders

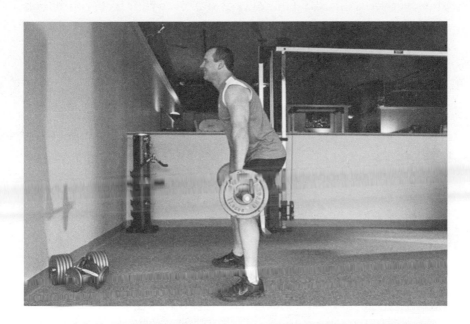

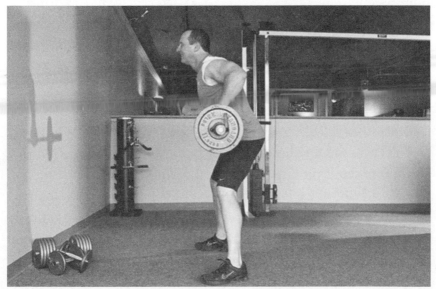

FIGURE 5.16 Barbell row. The start, above, and the finish, below.

stay over your knees and your knees stay over your feet. Your knees should never go in front of your feet, and your shoulders should never go in front of your knees. If either occurs, your center of gravity is in front of your feet and you'll feel yourself being pulled forward. This puts stress on your back, increasing the chance of injury. Keeping your back slightly arched while performing this exercise keeps the spine in its most protected position.

Raise the weight up along your legs until the bar touches your stomach, then return to the start position. Make sure you don't jerk the bar up and that your torso doesn't swing backward to gain momentum. Your torso shouldn't move during the exercise.

T-Bar Row: This exercise is a little easier than the barbell row. You place the weights on a bar affixed to the equipment, so stabilizing the weight is easier. The T-bar row machine comes in two styles: one is straight and the other has a 45-degree angle pad. I prefer the one with the 45-degree angle pad, because with the regular T-bar row machine, there's a much greater tendency to incorporate your legs into the lift. The one with the 45-degree angle places your feet off the floor, so there's no way your legs can help you lift the weight. They can only push against the foot plates to help you stabilize your torso.

The movement is similar to the barbell row. Hold the handles so your forearms pull up perpendicular to the floor. In the regular T-bar row, the stance is the same as for the barbell row. Stand very close to the T-bar row machine, so that, while performing the exercise, it runs very close to your thighs until it touches your stomach. The T-bar row machine with the angled pad has you resting on your chest. Position yourself so your chin is just off the end of the pad. Pull up so your forearms are pulling perpendicular to the floor. In both cases, you can start with a slight hunch in your back and complete with a slight arch in your back. This guarantees the fullest range of motion of the lats and teres major.

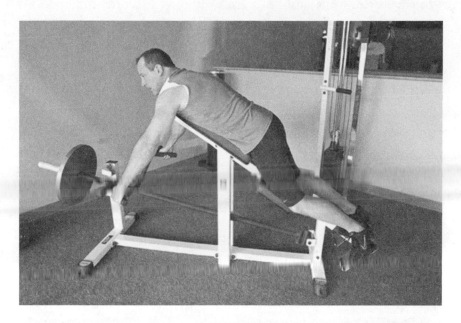

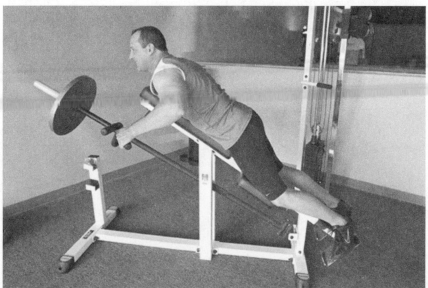

FIGURE 5.17 T-bar row. The start, above, and the finish, below.

One-Arm Row: If dumbbells are available, the one-arm row is a good choice. Here, you perform the row movement one side at a time. When you're working the right side, you place your left hand and left knee on the bench. Space your hand and knee so when they're supporting your weight, your back is parallel to the floor. Place your right foot farther back than your left knee and slightly wider than shoulder width from the bench. This gives you a strong base of support and good stability. Make sure your right foot is pointing forward and your right knee is slightly bent. You should feel yourself weight bearing evenly on your left hand, left knee, and right foot. Your back should be level with the floor, both horizontally and vertically. Start the exercise with your back slightly hunched. Raise the dumbbell by running your arm along your side until your elbow is slightly above your back. As you raise it, go from a slightly hunched to a slightly arched position, for the maximum range of motion. Return the dumbbell to the start position, making sure to not lock your elbow; keep it slightly bent. If you feel your torso twisting to the opposite side while performing the exercise, you're using too much weight. Your shoulders should stay level during the entire movement.

Biceps

The biceps runs from your elbow to your shoulder. At the elbow, the biceps attaches to a small protrusion in the *radius* bone of your forearm called the *biceps tuberosity*. From there, the biceps attaches to two locations at the shoulder. The short head of the biceps attaches to the *coracoid process* of the shoulder blade, and the long head attaches to the superior border of the glenoid fossa. This means that the long head actually passes through the shoulder joint (see Figure 5.19). Both heads attach down at a common tendon that connects to the elbow.

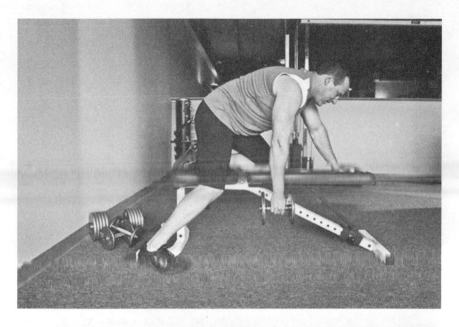

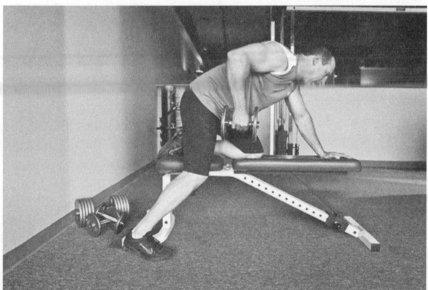

FIGURE 5.18 One-arm row. The start, above, and the finish, below.

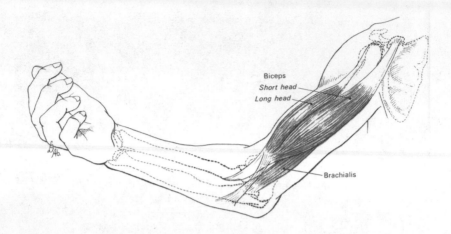

FIGURE 5.19 Biceps passing through shoulder joint.

The main function of the biceps is as an elbow flexor. This means that the biceps closes the elbow joint when you bring your hand palm up toward your shoulder while bending your elbow. Another function of the biceps is as a supinator. This is when you turn your palm from face down to face up.

When strengthening the biceps, focus on the muscle acting as an elbow flexor. Many exercise variations work the biceps. As long as you maintain the basic concept of elbow flexion, you can't go wrong—whether you do barbell or dumbbell curls, seated or standing. I like to do them seated, because then I can isolate the biceps without compensating with a lot of lower back sway. If you sway, you're losing efficiency by not fully using the biceps.

Biceps Curl: From a seated position with arms at your sides, curl one arm so you bring the dumbbell from the down position toward your shoulder. Make sure you bring it as close to directly in front of your shoulder as possible. The biceps is in the front of the upper arm, so you should bring the weight in front of you, not to the side of you.

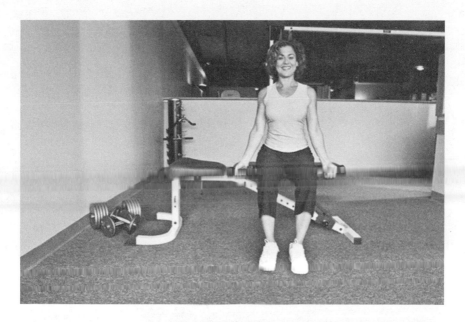

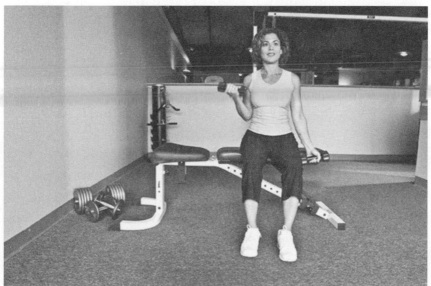

FIGURE 5.20 Biceps curl. The start, above, and the finish, below.

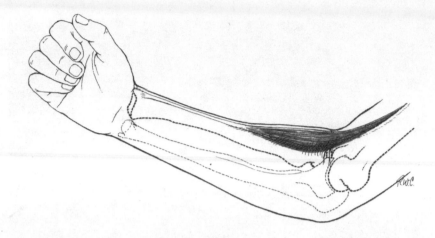

FIGURE 5.21 (a) Brachialis and (b) brachioradialis.

Make sure you get a full range of motion and keep your palm facing upward throughout the exercise. I've seen people starting the motion with their palms facing down and then twisting their palms until they're facing up. This is wrong. The biceps acts as the primary mover only when the palm is face up. When the palm is face down, the **brachialis** is the primary mover, and when the palm is halfway up, you're working the **brachioradialis** (see Figure 5.21). These are best worked through reverse curls, which we'll get to later. So if you twist your forearm, the biceps isn't doing the work through the entire range of motion. This is inefficient and won't yield maximum results. The biceps does twist the forearm, but only at a set position, not as you flex your elbow. These are two separate and distinct movements.

In addition, make sure your elbow isn't jammed into your side. Keep it at the side of your body. Let the shoulder and back musculature work naturally to stabilize your arm. Don't raise your elbow while performing the exercise. If you do, you're incorporating some shoulder musculature as a primary mover rather than a stabilizer. You're also shortening the biceps at both ends—at the elbow and the shoulder. This breaks a main rule of weight lifting, which is to shorten the muscle at one end while keeping the other end stable.

Once you've completely lowered the dumbbell in one hand, you can begin to raise the opposite hand. Keep alternating arms in this manner until you've completed your reps.

Preacher Curl: If you have a gym membership, the gym will likely have a preacher curl bench and an E-Z curl bar. You can perform this exercise instead of—or in addition to—the biceps curl. If you don't have a gym membership, the biceps curl is sufficient. In the preacher curl, grip the bar so your hands are shoulder width apart. Your upper arm should hang over the bench. Start with your elbow extended up to just before it locks. Then, lift the weight until your forearms are just beyond perpendicular to the floor. Slowly

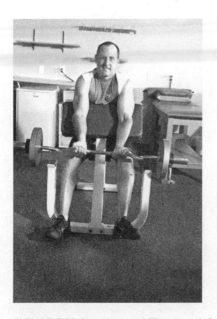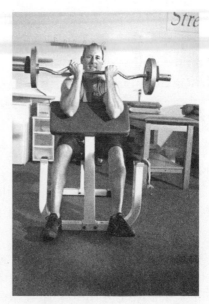

FIGURE 5.22 Preacher curl. The start, left, and the finish, right.

return to the start position and continue through the repetitions in
this fashion.

The most difficult element of this exercise is finding the right
position on the bench and maintaining it throughout the set. You
don't want to hang over the bench, because then you're bringing
your shoulders too far forward. This greatly reduces the muscle's
range of motion, causing you to lose some efficiency. If you lean
back too far, you end up using your body to lift the weight as you
drop down into the seat. This is also inefficient.

To find the right position, first sit in the seat. Lift the armrest
until your back is perpendicular to the floor, while your arms hang
over the armrest. Now, lift the bar up until you're seated. Slide
your feet under the bench. This will help stabilize your torso and
keep you in a good lifting position. As you lower the bar, make
sure that bringing the weight down doesn't bring you forward. If
you can't control your body's movement, you need to reduce the
weight.

Keep in mind that the biceps is a very small muscle in relation
to the other muscles in your body. The biceps is very limited in its
motion, so you don't need more than one or two exercises to isolate it. Often, people devote too much energy to the biceps. You're
better off spending more time working the bigger muscle groups.

Reverse Curl: Here's where we isolate the brachialis, located between the biceps and the triceps and the brachioradialis, located
in the forearm. For the bodybuilder, this completes the elbow region by filling out the side of the arm. If you're just looking for
function, it allows you to lift things more easily, even when your
palms are facing down.

Typically, you perform the exercise standing, either with a
straight bar or an E-Z curl bar. You don't have to worry about swaying, because the muscles are so small (and therefore, the weight
so low), that you won't have much difficulty stabilizing the body.

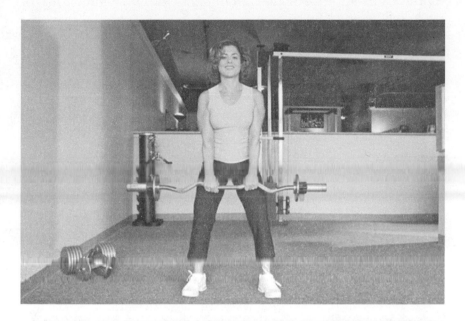

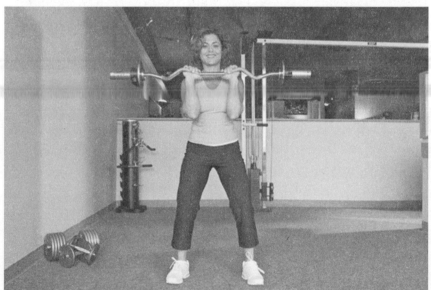

FIGURE 5.23 Reverse curl. The start, above, and the finish, below.

Stand with your feet shoulder width apart and your knees slightly bent. Hold the bar with your hands shoulder width apart, with a hand overgrip so your palms are facing down. Keeping your elbows at your sides, slowly raise the bar until it reaches your chest and then return it to the start position. The range of motion should be about 150 degrees, similar to range used in the biceps curl.

Forearms

The forearm is comprised of the wrist extensors, which bend your wrist toward the back of your hand, and the wrist flexors, which bend your wrist toward your palm. They're typically strengthened by acting as stabilizers during other exercises, so most people don't take the time to isolate them. But if you perform an activity that requires repetitive motion for long periods of time, such as hammering, typing, tennis, or golf, I highly recommend strengthening these muscles. If your forearm muscles are weak, you could develop carpal tunnel syndrome or tennis elbow as a result of these activities. You'd typically add this group at the end of the biceps workout.

Wrist Curl: You can do these with either dumbbells or a barbell; dumbbells are easier. For the wrist flexors, hold the weight in your hand with your palm facing up at the end of a table or bench. Support your forearm so only your wrist hangs off the end. To keep your forearm on the support, hold it with your other hand. Slowly lower the weight as your wrist bends backward. You should be able to reach about 90 degrees of motion. Now, slowly lift the weight until your wrist is fully flexed forward—about 80 degrees. Continue the motion in this fashion.

For wrist extension, place your forearm on the support, with your palm facing down. Again, have just your wrist and hand off the support. Perform the exercise the same way as the wrist flexion,

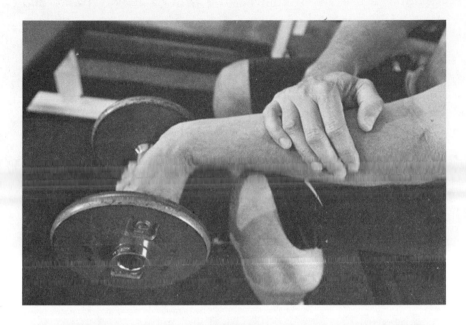

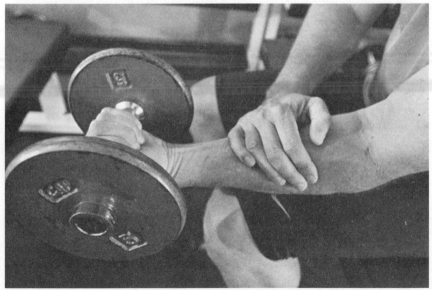

FIGURE 5.24 Wrist curl (flexion and extension). The start, above, and the finish, below.

lowering the weight by allowing the wrist to flex downward and then raising the wrist upward to full range. You'll always be able to lift more weight with the wrist flexors, so don't try to lift as much with the extensors.

Rope Curl: To build a little muscular endurance, run a very small weight through a rope and attach the rope at both ends of a broomstick. Hold the broomstick with your palms facing up and your hands shoulder width apart. Your elbows will be at your side and bent to 90 degrees, and the weight will be centered between your hands. Try to roll your wrists under to roll the rope over the broomstick and bring the weight up. Then allow it to go down again. Do that several times, and then do just the opposite and roll your wrists over to work the other muscle group. This builds the muscular endurance of both the extensor and flexor groups because it focuses more on sustaining contraction than resistance. This is probably a more functional exercise for the forearm muscles, because they act primarily as stabilizers of the wrist during most activities—rarely as primary movers. In this case, combining the rope curl with the wrist curls is a good combination.

The Thigh

Our leg exercises work the muscles of the thighs, hips, and lower leg. The upper leg muscles including the thighs and hips are the easiest to understand, so we'll start there.

Squats, lunges, and straight-leg dead lifts, which work the upper leg, or thigh, incorporate most of the muscle groups of the thigh and hip. You can also perform isolated exercises to strengthen the individual muscle groups of the thighs and hips.

Squat: This is the best overall exercise for the entire body but most importantly for the entire leg. Many consider it dangerous, but

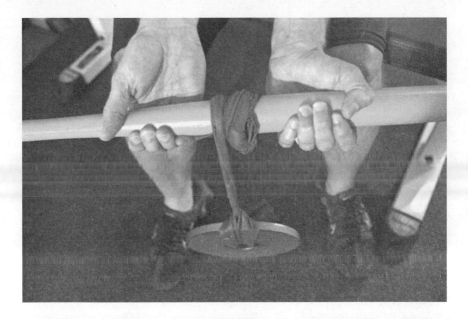

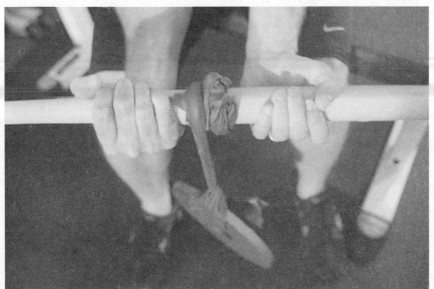

FIGURE 5.25 Rope curl (flexion and extension). The start, above, and the finish, below.

if done correctly, it's the most effective way of strengthening the entire leg, especially the quadriceps, glutes, and hamstrings. It also represents the proper position for lifting objects. To learn the squat as an exercise is to learn to lift properly. Every knee patient I work with learns the squat as part of his or her therapy regimen.

A squat is not to be confused with a deep knee bend. In a deep knee bend, you align your shoulders, hips, and ankles so your knees come forward. When performing the squat, the shoulder, knee, and ankle all stay in alignment through the entire range of motion, providing a better mechanical advantage for your quadriceps, the strongest muscle in the body. This offers the greatest opportunity to create force and lift more weight.

The knee is a modified hinge joint, designed to stay in one position as the upper and lower leg move around it, as in a squat. It can't take the sheer force that a deep knee bend places on it. It should come as no surprise when knee injuries result as the knee moves forward while performing a squat. The way to exercise safely and effectively is to stress the muscles, not the joints. Of all the weight-lifting exercises in this book, the squat requires the greatest amount of balance, so it's a good idea to practice the form of the squat without weight before moving on to lifting resistance.

For your starting position, place your feet slightly wider than shoulder width apart. This can vary depending on the length of your leg, so experiment to find the most comfortable position that allows a full range of motion but still keeps your knees over your heels. The wider apart your feet are, the easier it is to allow your buttocks to go all the way back through the full range of motion without having your knees go forward. Pointing your toes slightly outward helps as well.

The next thing to consider is whether you'll be holding dumbbells or a barbell. If you use a barbell, you'll hold it on your shoulders; you'll keep dumbbells at your sides.

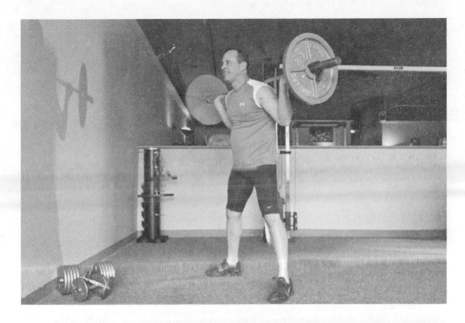

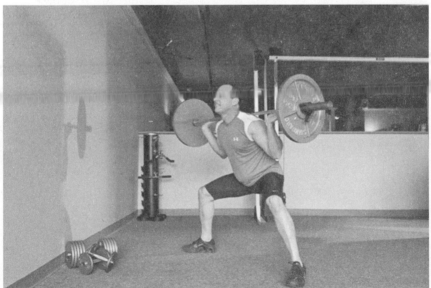

FIGURE 5.26 Squat. The start, above, and the finish, below.

To begin the exercise, pretend that you're going to sit in a chair and place your buttocks at the back of the seat. Your buttocks lead the motion. As your buttocks move back, your shoulders remain over your knees. The only way to achieve this is to begin arching your back. For some people, this is a concern because there is a misconception that arching your back could cause an injury, but as you arch your back, the muscles that run along your spine contract to pull the bones of your spine into a locked position. This makes the spine act as one integral unit instead of many independent bones, limiting the chance of injuring any structures surrounding it. It's now recognized that the spine should be in an arched position when lifting objects.

Continue lowering your buttocks until your thighs are parallel to the floor. You should be weight bearing mostly on your heels throughout the exercise. If you're on the balls of your feet, you're shifting the emphasis of the exercise from the quadriceps to the calf. Your shoulders should be over your knees and ankles, your chest should be forward, and you should be looking either forward or up. Once your thighs are parallel to the floor, slowly begin to return to the start position.

Because of the difficulty in maintaining your balance and proper form while still reaching the full range of motion, you may find yourself breaking form to reach the full range of motion. This is inefficient and potentially harmful. You're better off going through a shorter range of motion but keeping good form. As your balance improves, you'll be able to fully extend your range of motion so your thighs are parallel to the floor. Once you can do this while maintaining control and good balance, you can add resistance to enhance the value of the exercise. Tight muscles might hinder your ability to perform a proper squat by limiting your range of motion. Proper stretching, which you'll read about in the next chapter, can remedy this.

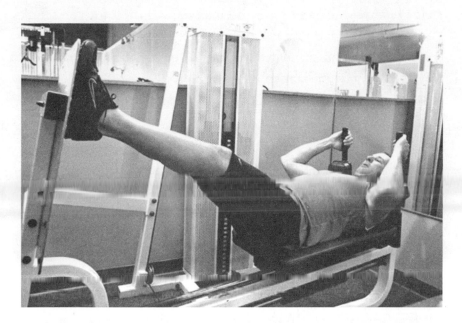

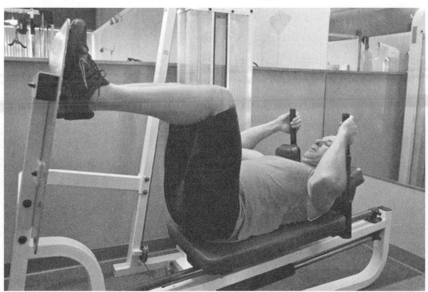

FIGURE 5.27 Leg press. The start, above, and the finish, below.

Leg Press: If you don't have the balance required for the squat, and you have a gym membership, the leg press is another general thigh exercise that simulates a squat. The problem with it is that you can't keep your back in an arched position, and arched is the best lifting position for the back. For this reason, I don't recommend lifting maximum weights on the leg press. You should also limit the range of motion to a 90-degree knee bend. This limits how much the lower back rounds, so it can't enter an unstable position.

To start, place your feet on the platform of the leg press so the lower leg is perpendicular to the platform. Your feet should be hip width apart, and your hips, knees, and feet should be in alignment. Start to straighten your legs by pushing through your heels. This doesn't mean you should take the balls of your feet off the platform; just focus most of your force through your heels. Stop just before your knees lock, and slowly return to the start position, which is with your legs at just short of a 90-degree angle.

Straight-Leg Dead Lift: This exercise works the glutes and hamstrings, and, like the squat, it's also misunderstood. Many consider it dangerous because it puts a lot of stress on the back. That's true only if it's done incorrectly. In fact, this is one of the mainstay exercises I use with most, if not all, of my back patients.

Weak glutes and hamstrings can cause the muscles of the lower back to overwork, and eventually they break down, causing chronic problems in that region. Strong glutes and hamstrings take pressure off the lower back muscles and allow them to function normally. Another benefit of this exercise is that it lifts a sagging butt. There is no better exercise for strengthening your buttocks than the straight-leg dead lift.

When done correctly, the glutes and hamstrings pull at the hip to raise your torso. The lower back muscles simply stabilize the torso, transferring the weight from your arms to your legs. This

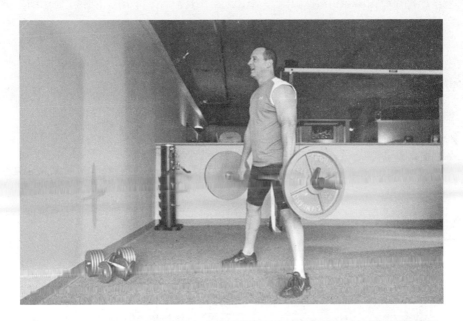

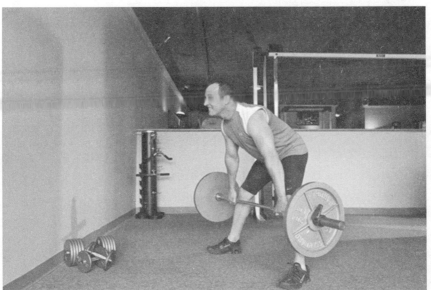

FIGURE 5.28 Straight-leg dead lift. The start, above, and the finish, below.

reinforces the goal of lifting with your legs and only activating the lower back muscles to stabilize the torso.

You can perform the straight-leg dead lift using either dumbbells or a barbell. Stand with your feet slightly more than shoulder width apart and your toes pointed slightly out. Hold dumbbells in front of your thighs, or grab a barbell at a position slightly wider than shoulder width. In either case, your palms should be facing your thighs, your knees slightly bent, your back slightly arched, and your elbows straight throughout the entire motion. You should be weight bearing on your heels, but your toes shouldn't come off the floor.

Slowly bring the weight down your legs, keeping it as close to your legs as possible through the entire motion. This is where most people lose the form. If you allow the weight to come forward, you're forcing your lower back muscles to support this load and you are setting yourself up for injury. You never want the lower back muscles to do anything but stabilize the torso. As you bring the weight down, your butt should be moving backward. This offsets the movement of your torso in front of your legs and limits any excessive weight from ending up in front of your feet. Make sure all the motion occurs at the hip.

Continue lowering the weight down the front of your legs until you begin to feel a pull in the hamstrings. This will vary for each individual. You don't have to reach the floor. Some people can do this while maintaining good form, while others may be able to go no farther than just below the knees. The important thing is to keep good form. The distance you travel will increase as you become more accustomed to performing the exercise. If you reach the floor and still don't feel a pull in your hamstrings, something is probably wrong with your form: either your back is hunched or you're bending too much at the knee. Try to make these corrections and see if you feel the stretch at the end range. Once you do, begin to return to the start position.

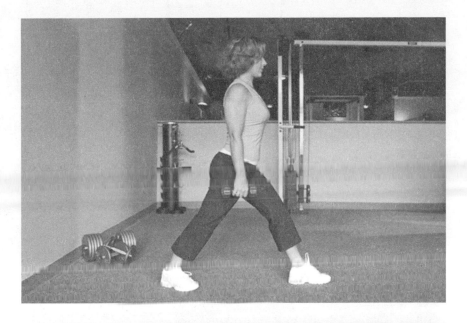

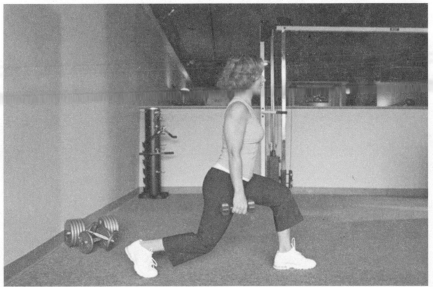

FIGURE 5.29 Lunge. The start, above, and the finish, below.

Lunge: The lunge is relatively easy because it doesn't require much flexibility or balance. You can use dumbbells or a barbell. Hold dumbbells at your sides and a barbell on your shoulders. With your feet shoulder width apart and pointing forward, place one foot in front of the other at a comfortable distance. If you feel off-balance, widen your stance.

To start, you'll come up on the ball of your back foot, keeping your back upright throughout the motion. Drop your back knee toward the floor. Most people think of lunging as a forward motion, and what typically happens is that the front knee moves forward in front of the foot. The key to success with this exercise is to keep your knee directly above your front foot, not in front of it. Continue to drop the back knee down until it's just above the floor, still making sure your back is upright and not bent forward. Once you've achieved this, slowly bring yourself back up to the starting position. Make sure you raise yourself by pushing through the heel of your front foot. This ensures you're using the quadriceps of the front leg as the primary mover. At the top of the motion, make sure you don't lock your knees. You can perform the exercise either by alternating feet after each set or by doing three sets on one foot and then three sets on the other foot.

Abduction: Although the quads, glutes, and hamstrings are the primary movers in squats, dead lifts, and lunges, you're also activating the adductors and abductors (inner and outer thigh muscles, respectively) as stabilizers of the pelvis while performing these exercises. If you have time and are concerned about isolating these two stabilizer muscles, you can perform additional exercises.

You can perform this exercise lying down with cuff weights on your ankles or with a pulley system. For the former, place the cuff weights on your ankles and lie down on either your right side or your left side. To perform the abduction, bend the knee of the leg on the bottom for additional balance and stability. Lock the

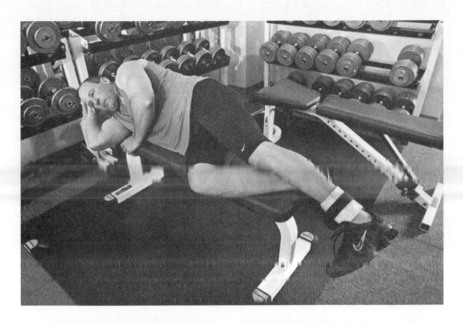

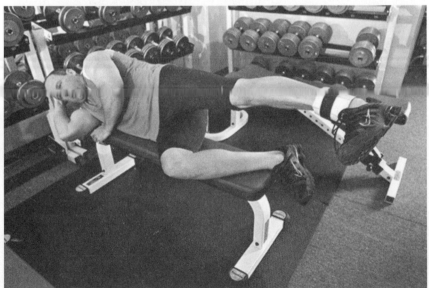

FIGURE 5.30 Abduction. The start, above, and the finish, below.

knee of the top leg and flex your foot. Raise your top leg to hip height, making sure it's in line with your torso. A common mistake is bringing your leg in front of your torso, which forces your hip flexors to perform part of the exercise. Slowly bring your leg down to the start position.

If you use the pulley system, attach the pulley to your ankle with an ankle strap. Stand so the leg you're working is farthest from the pulley. You may need to stand with your nonworking leg on a platform or weight so that the foot of your working leg can clear the floor. Bend the knee of the nonworking leg, keeping it above your foot. Lock the knee of the working leg. Flex your toes and pull the leg out to the side. There are about 40 degrees of hip abduction motion; beyond that you begin to side bend using your lower back muscles on the side you are performing the exercise, so don't pull to the point where you begin to bend your torso to the side. Your torso should remain upright and stable throughout the motion. Return to the starting position, making sure the leg is in line with the torso when performing the exercise.

Adduction: For the adductor, start the exercise by lying on your side. Place the foot of your top leg in front of the knee of your bottom leg. The foot of your top leg will be flat on the floor to give you a point to push through to support yourself. Lock the knee of your bottom leg and flex your foot. Now, raise this leg up, keeping your thigh in line with your torso. Keep in mind that this is a very small motion of only 10 or 20 degrees. Return to the starting position. I use this exercise in therapy quite often, because it requires almost no equipment and very little balance.

To use the pulley system, attach the strap to the ankle of the leg closest to the machine. Again, you may have to stand on a platform or weight to allow the foot of the moving leg to clear the floor. Place the foot of the nonworking leg slightly farther than shoulder width from the working leg, to give yourself some range

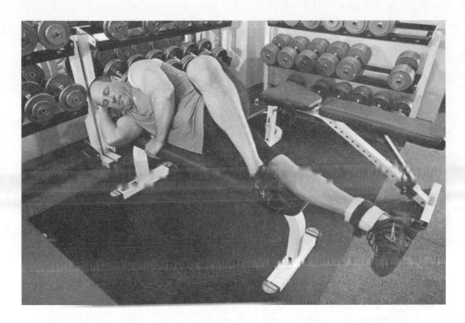

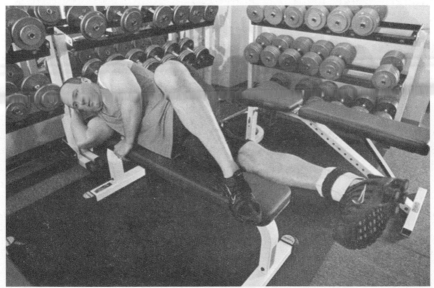

FIGURE 5.31 Adduction. The start, above, and the finish, below.

to work with. Bend the knee of the outside leg and lock the knee of the moving leg. With toes flexed, bring the foot toward the opposite leg until it passes in front of it. Return it to the start position.

In both adduction and abduction, you're putting some stress on the leg supporting you, so expect to feel the front thigh and hip abductors of the leg that is supporting you working. If you feel pain in the knee of the leg supporting you, your knee is likely in front of your foot. Be sure to keep your knee directly above your foot.

Extension: If you want to isolate the muscles of the upper leg, you can do extensions and hamstring curls. Typically performed on a leg extension machine, extensions isolate the quadriceps. To set the machine correctly, position the seat back so your knee is in line with the pivot point of the machine, and position the foot cushion so it aligns with your ankle. Flex your feet when performing the exercise, and make sure you go through the full range of motion. In addition, keep your back hunched to lengthen the quadriceps and achieve the longest range possible.

Hamstring Curl: You can do hamstring curls standing, seated, or lying down, but you will need a piece of equipment. The machines vary from gym to gym, but regardless of the equipment, the alignments are the same. Position the knee so it's in line with the pivot point of the device, and position the foot cushion so it aligns with the top of the heel. Flex your foot and make sure you go through the full range of motion. Keeping your back in an arched position gives your hamstrings maximum range.

The Calf

The calf, located behind the shin, has two muscle components: the *soleus* and the gastrocnemius. The soleus extends from the Achilles tendon to the two lower bones of the shin. The function

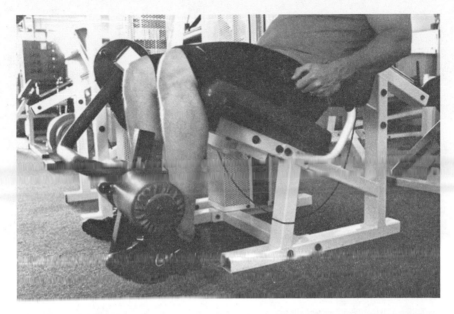

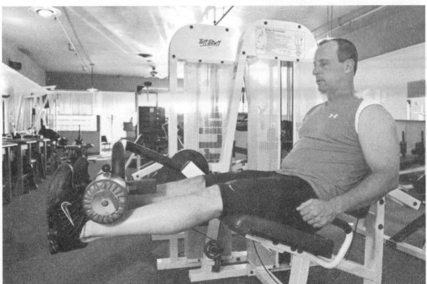

FIGURE 5.32 Extension. The start, above, and the finish, below.

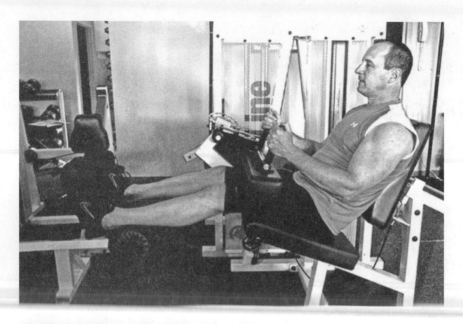

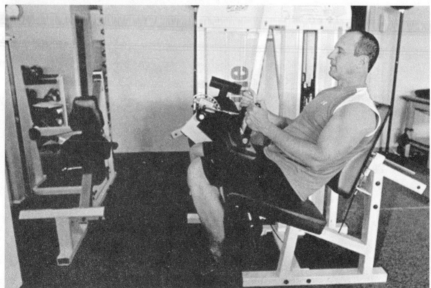

FIGURE 5.33 Hamstring curl. The start, above, and the finish, below.

of this muscle, which doesn't go beyond the knee, is to plantar flex—or raise—the heel. The gastrocnemius also attaches at the Achilles tendon, but it passes the knee joint and extends up the femur. This muscle plantar flexes the ankle but also can flex the knee joint.

Calf Raise: The most effective exercise for the soleus is the calf raise, and you can perform it using any type of equipment. You can even do it while seated. Just place a weight along your knees and raise your heels up while pushing down on the balls of your feet. Just make sure you go through the full range of motion. If you're using a seated calf raise machine, place the balls of your feet at the end of the footrest and place the weight support over your thighs. With the cushion across your thighs, take the weight off the stand. Allow your heels to be controlled down to where you begin to feel a stretch in the calf or Achilles tendon. Then, raise your heels up as far as you can, again going through the full range of motion.

If your natural body type is such that you need more strengthening on one side of the calf than the other, alter the position of your feet. Normally, you'd point your toes forward. To work the inside of your calf, point your toes outward a little. For the outside of your

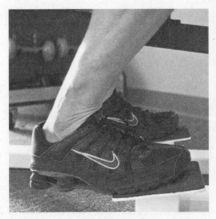 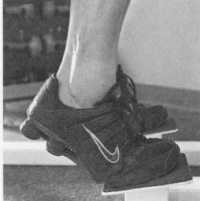

FIGURE 5.34 Calf raise. The start, left, and the finish, right.

calf, point your toes inward. This is mostly for aesthetics; novices should keep the foot pointed forward.

Donkey Calf: To strengthen the gastrocnemius, you need to keep the knee straight throughout the exercise. You can perform this exercise using any piece of equipment—a donkey calf raise machine, a standing calf machine, a leg press, even the edge of a stair—as long as you're able to keep your knees straight. My favorite is the donkey calf machine, because it places the weight right on the pelvis. This prevents the spine from transmitting the weight down to the pelvis and finally to the legs, which could strain your lower back.

One mistake many people make when trying to keep their knees straight is *hyperextending* them. If your knees bow backward even slightly, correct the position by straightening them out. Hyperextension can cause knee pain by irritating the underside of the kneecap.

Plantarflexion: If a machine is not available to strengthen the calf, the use of a elastic ribbon can suffice. To start the exercise, have your leg raised off a support such as a table, chair or even the floor with a bolster or pillow. This allows the ankle to move through range of motion without the heel catching. Your toes will be pointing toward your face. Slowly move your ankle so that your toes are pointing away from you. To complete the exercise, slowly move your ankle so you are at the start position. The elastic ribbons are sold with different resistances. This allows progression of resistance to occur even with this device. The resistance ribbon should be placed so it runs across the balls of the foot.

Toe Raise: In front of the shin is a muscle called the anterior tibialis, which is responsible for dorsiflexing, or weight bearing on your heels by raising the front of your foot. This muscle attaches

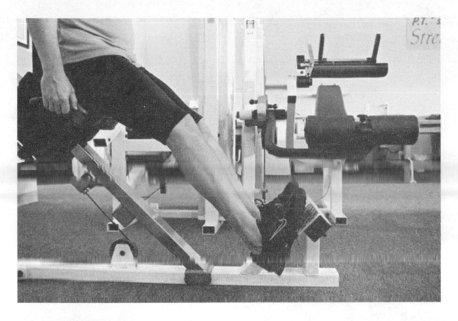

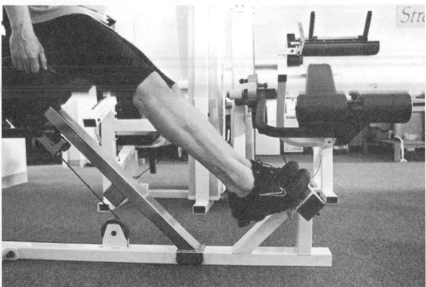

FIGURE 5.35 Donkey calf. The start, above, and the finish, below.

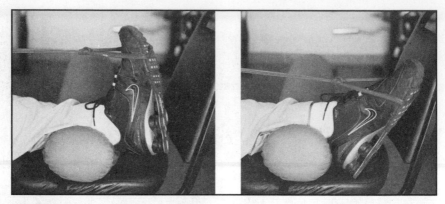

FIGURE 5.36 Plantarflexion

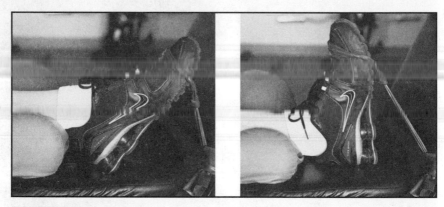

FIGURE 5.37 Dorsiflexion

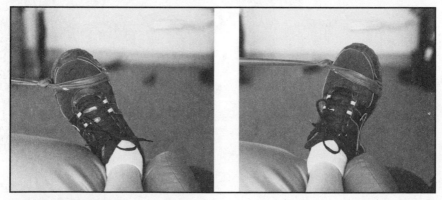

FIGURE 5.38 Inversion

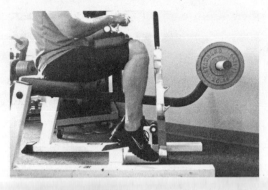

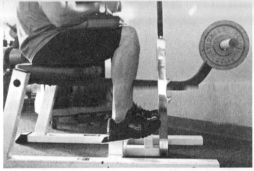

FIGURE 5.39 Toe raise. The start, above, and the finish, below.

at one end to several of the bones on the bottom of the foot and at the other end to the lateral portion of the tibia, a bone in the lower leg. If your gym doesn't have the equipment for this exercise, you can use a seated calf machine. Instead of the balls of the feet, place your heel on the footrest. Now instead of raising your heels, raise the toes and balls of your feet. If this is too difficult, simply stand with your heels on the edge of a stair. Make sure you have good support and raise and lower the balls of your feet and toes. This is a very small muscle and requires little resistance. You should be able to strengthen it using only your body weight as resistance.

Dorsiflexion: An alternative exercise to toe raises to strengthen the anterior tibialis is dorsiflexion with a theraband (elastic ribbon that can be used to create resistance). The ankle is raised off the surface that is supporting the lower leg by placing a bolster or pillow under the ankle. This allows the ankle to go through range of motion without having the heel catching on the surface. The exercise starts with the toes pointing away from your face. Slowly bend your ankle as your toes move toward you until you can not move any farther. In most cases, this point is slightly beyond when your foot is perpendicular to the ground. To finish, slowly return your foot to the start point. Make sure that when you are at the start point, you are not feeling a straining in the anterior tibialis. The resistance ribbon should be place in line with the base of the toes, not on the toes themselves.

Inversion: The muscles that support the inner portion of the ankle as well as helps to support the arch of the foot are the anterior and posterior tibialis muscles. The movement that these two muscles create when they contract is called inversion. The movement consists of rotating your foot from facing outside to facing inward. Start with the leg being supported on a surface with a bolster or pillow to allow the ankle motion to occur without the heel catching on the surface. The toes will be facing outward to the side of the body. Slowly move the ankle to the foot is pointing inward. Slowly return the foot to the starting position to complete the exercise. Make sure that at the starting position that there is not too much of a pull to create a strain of the posterior tibialis. The resistance ribbon should be placed so it runs across the balls of the foot.

Eversion: The muscles that support the outer ankle are called the peroneous muscles. The movement they create when contracted is called eversion. This motion consists of starting with your foot pointing inward and then being moved to point outward toward the side of the body. To start the exercise, place the leg on a support with a bolster or pillow under the ankle so the ankle can go

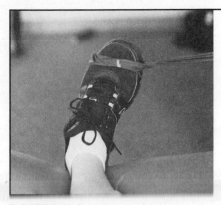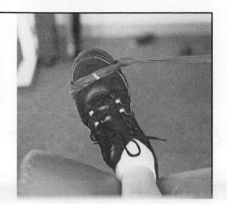

FIGURE 5.40 Eversion

through motion with the heel catching on the surface. The toes will be facing inward toward the middle of the body. Slowing turn the foot out pointing the toes to the side of the body. Slowly return to the start position to complete the exercise. The resistance ribbon should be placed so that it runs across the balls of the foot.

The Shoulders

The muscles of the shoulder, known as the deltoid, attach at the humerus, or upper arm bone, and the deltoid tuberosity, a long protuberance on the side of the upper arm bone. The three elements of the deltoid are the anterior, medial, and posterior head. The anterior head attaches from the deltoid tuberosity to the lateral third of the collarbone, as well as around the anterior portion of the acromium process, a component of the shoulder blade. The lateral head attaches from the deltoid tuberosity to the lateral aspect of the acromium process. The posterior head attaches from the deltoid tuberosity to the spine of the shoulder blade (see Figure 5.41).

The deltoid assists in abduction of the arm, which involves raising the arm out to the side of the body and continuing over

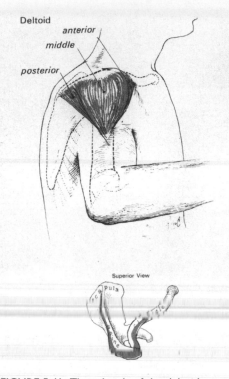

FIGURE 5.41: Three heads of the deltoids.

the head. A muscle that assists in this action is the supraspinatus, which attaches to the back of the shoulder blade and runs to the upper portion of the arm bone. For basic weight training, you don't need to isolate and strengthen these two muscles independently; you can work both during the course of the following deltoid exercises.

Military Press: The basic exercise for the deltoid is the military press. It strengthens the three heads of the deltoid as one integral unit, and you can perform it with either dumbbells or a barbell. You can bring the barbell down either in front of the body or behind the neck, but when bringing it behind the neck there's a tendency to move your elbows behind the line of your shoulders,

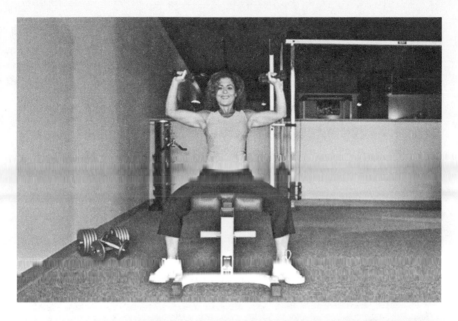

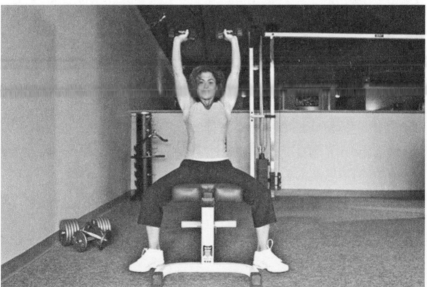

FIGURE 5.42 Military press. The start, above, and the finish, below.

and this puts stress on the front of the shoulder. By driving the arm bone forward, you can pinch tendons and stress ligaments and the joint capsule, creating a potential for injury. It's safer to bring the bar down in front of your body. Better yet, use dumbbells. They make it easier for you to keep your elbows either in perfect alignment with your shoulders or slightly in front. This way, there's no chance of injury to the front of your shoulder.

You can perform the military press either standing or seated. Seated offers more stability and less chance of incorporating other muscle groups. It also reduces the chance of arching the lower back too much, which could cause injury. When performing the seated military press, you need to keep your buttocks against the back support. The two points of contact are the shoulders and buttocks. You should maintain a normal arch in the back. This is the safest and most efficient position for the lower back when lifting. If you're lifting heavy resistance, wear a weight-lifting belt, which transmits the resistance from the rib cage to the pelvis. Because there's no bony support between these areas, the muscles that stabilize the torso, including those of the lower back, have to work very hard. If you lift heavy weights, you increase the chance of straining these muscles if you don't wear a weight-lifting belt.

Starting with the weights at shoulder height and palms facing forward, begin to lift them overhead. Your feet should be shoulder width apart and flat on the floor, for good support and balance, and your hands should stay over your elbows throughout the motion. Because your shoulder attaches to your upper arm, which ends at your elbow, the weight must remain over your elbow to push directly against the resistance. Keep your head against the backrest. This keeps your neck in good alignment and the weights from moving in front of the line of your shoulders. Raise the weights until your elbows are just short of locking. Because your elbows will move in toward your head as you lift them, the weights will move closer together. This doesn't mean they should touch, and

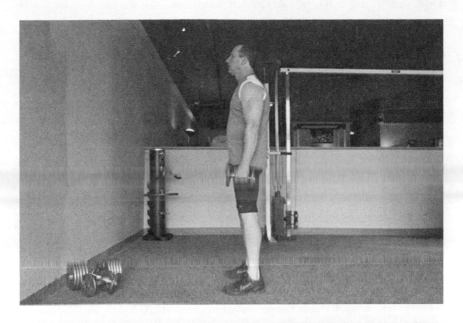

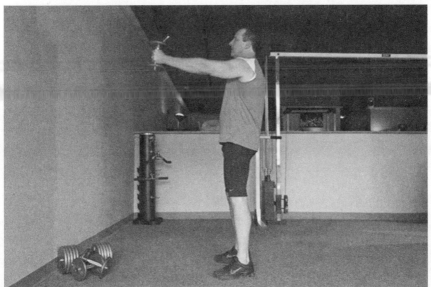

FIGURE 5.43 Front lateral. The start, above, and the finish, below.

they certainly shouldn't clank together. Slowly return the weights to the point where your elbows are just below the line of your shoulders. Your elbows don't have to come down and touch your sides on every repetition.

Eventually, you might progress to the point where you are using such heavy weights that you can no longer raise the weights from the floor to shoulder height. To accomplish this now, you will have to incorporate your legs to get the weight from the floor to your knees, then to shoulder height. To reach the start position, begin by placing the dumbbells on your knees. One leg at a time, quickly raise your knees to build enough momentum to elevate the weights to shoulder height. You do this to reserve all your shoulder energy for the exercise. Taking the weights from the floor to shoulder height requires a lot of energy and makes the exercise less efficient. Also, as you progress, you might get to a point where you can no longer swing the weights from your sides to shoulder height.

Next, you can isolate the three heads of the deltoid individually. If you have time constraints, focus on the posterior deltoid. Because we lift things in front of our bodies, we use the anterior and, to a lesser degree, lateral deltoid more often than the posterior deltoid. This can create a muscle imbalance. Many shoulder injuries result from this imbalance, because it alters the mechanics of the shoulder joint. At a minimum, you should isolate the posterior deltoid so it remains as strong as the anterior and lateral deltoid.

Front Lateral: To perform a front lateral, you raise your arms from your sides in front of you to the point where your hands are just below shoulder height Using dumbbells to perform this exercise gives you better control than a barbell. They prevent your stronger arm from overtaking your weaker arm and performing more of the exercise. Hold the dumbbells in front of your thighs. Keep your feet shoulder width apart, with knees slightly bent. Elbows are very slightly bent, and palms are facing downward. Either one at a time or together, raise the dumbbells straight out in front of you to just below shoulder height. Unlike other exercises, in this one, you inhale as you lift the weights. The reason you do the opposite with the front, side, and posterior lateral exercises is because inhaling raises the rib cage as you lift the weights. This keeps good contact between the upper arm bone and shoulder joint. Make sure the weights don't bring you onto your toes as you lift. If they do, you're probably lifting too much weight. Stay back on your heels throughout the exercise. Slowly return the weights back to the start position in front of your thighs.

Side Lateral: Side laterals are basically the same as front laterals, except you lift the dumbbell from the side of your body out to the side, to just below shoulder height. Palms are facing down, elbows are very slightly bent, and knees are bent. Doing one arm at a time is best, because you can hold onto a support with the other hand to stabilize yourself. Remember to inhale while raising the weights for this exercise.

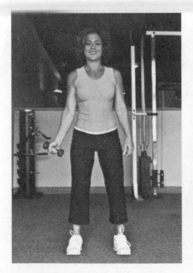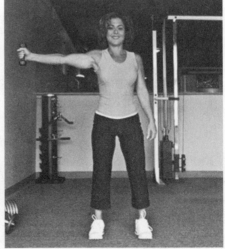

FIGURE 5.44: Side lateral. The start, left, and the finish, right.

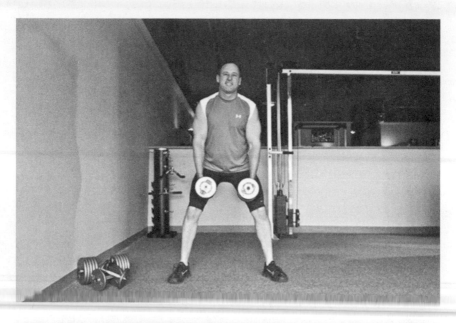

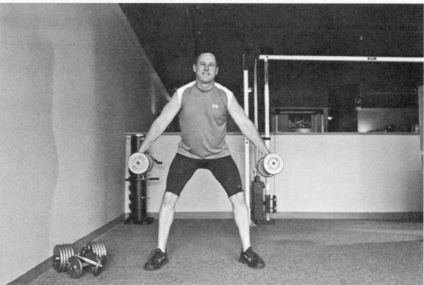

FIGURE 5.45 Posterior lateral. The start, above, and the finish, below.

Posterior Lateral: This exercise isolates the posterior deltoids and is crucial because the anterior deltoid has a natural tendency to be stronger than the posterior deltoid. With muscle imbalance comes improper posture and ultimately dysfunction and symptoms such as pain at the shoulder or neck. Many people don't understand the posterior lateral and perform it in potentially harmful positions. The proper technique is to stand with your feet slightly wider than shoulder width apart. Bend your knees and stick your buttocks back, making sure your knees stay over your heels. You should be weight bearing on your heels. Keep your back slightly arched and your shoulders over your feet throughout the motion. Hold the dumbbells in front of you, with your palms facing and your elbows bent very slightly. Slowly raise the weights out to your sides, keeping them on an arc very close to your body. The motion occurs from the shoulder, so you should not increase the bend in your elbow. The range of motion in this case is much less than most people think. You should come out only about 60 degrees from the centerline of your body. If you go farther, you'll begin to feel your shoulder blades coming together. This means you're now working the muscles between your shoulder blades and not the posterior deltoid. The range should stop just when you feel your shoulder blades begin to move inward toward each other. Slowly return the weights to the start position.

When performing the front lateral and side lateral, stop the range of motion just below shoulder height. This isolates the range of motion being performed to that created by the deltoid. Beyond this range, other muscles are performing the motion and efficacy is lost.

Shrugs: Everyone should perform shrugs, even novices. Shrugs work the upper *trapezius* muscles, which attach the arm, shoulder, shoulder blade, and collarbone to the spine. The trapezius are the main

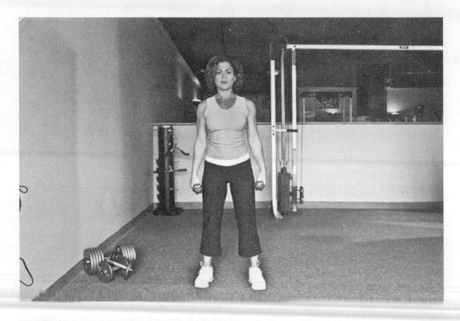

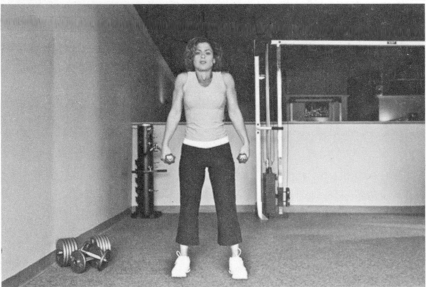

FIGURE 5.46 Shrugs. The start, above, and the finish, below.

muscles that support these bony structures, and it's common for them to tighten from overuse and cause muscle-tension headaches.

The exercise, which you perform standing with knees slightly bent, is simple and quick, and you can use a barbell or dumbbells. You hold a barbell in front of you against your thighs, and you hold dumbbells against the outside of your thighs. Keep your feet a little wider than shoulder width apart, your elbows straight, and your shoulders over your heels through the motion. Your back should remain in a normally arched position, and you should weight bear through your heels. Slowly raise the weight by bringing your shoulders up to your ears. Do not rotate forward or back; just come straight up. Breathe in on the way up to raise the rib cage in the direction of the exercise. Slowly return the weight to the start position.

External Rotation: The rotator cuff sits deep, under the deltoid in the shoulder. It is responsible for keeping the upper arm bone in the shoulder socket when performing activities. The exercise for strengthening this muscle group can be performed with dumbbells. Sit on a stool or a bench adjacent to a table. Place your elbow on the table so your upper arm is pointing to just below 90 degrees. Hold your elbow at 90 degrees through the whole motion. Start with your forearm pointed about 20 degrees below parallel to the floor and raise the weight until your forearm is pointing about 20 degrees above parallel. The total motion of this exercise is only about 40 degrees. Make sure you maintain a straight, sitting posture with your chest out and your shoulders pulled back.

The Triceps

The triceps has three heads that attach along the upper arm bone, the shaft of the upper arm bone, and the lower portion of the shoulder joint. The three heads join to a common tendon and attach

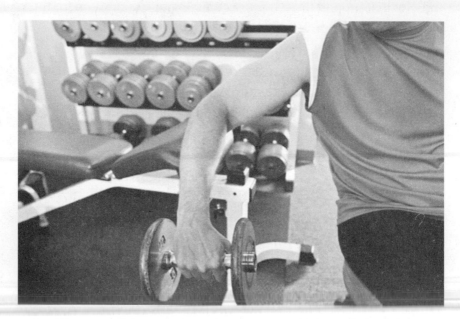

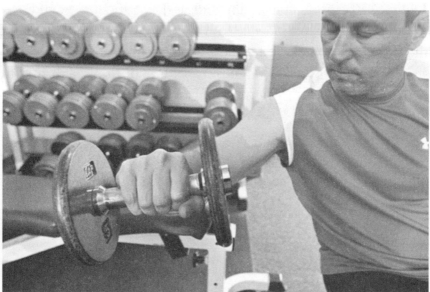

FIGURE 5.47 Rotator cuff. The start, above, and the finish, below.

at the elbow. The triceps' main function is to extend or straighten the elbow. Many exercises strengthen the triceps, but because it's a small muscle, select two or, at most, three exercises.

French Curl: My favorite triceps exercise is the French curl or, as many people know it, the skull crusher. Don't let the name scare you. It's a very safe exercise and the most efficient at isolating and strengthening the triceps. The exercise is typically performed with an E-Z curl bar, but you can also use dumbbells or a barbell. Lie on a bench with your feet flat on the floor and a little more than hip width apart for good stability. Grip the bar above your head, with your arms perpendicular to the floor, your hands shoulder width apart, and your thumbs on the same side of the bar as your fingers so you don't grip the bar too tightly. Slowly lower the bar to your forehead, making sure your elbows point straight up throughout the motion. Also make sure your elbows remain close to your body, and don't move laterally. Your wrists should stay straight; don't allow them to flex one way or the other, because this can irritate your wrist or forearm. Once the weights approach your forehead, return to the start position, to the point just before you lock your elbows.

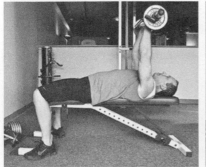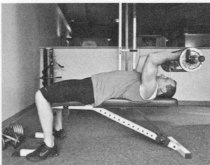

FIGURE 5.48 French curl. The start, left, and the finish, right.

Triceps Extension: This exercise is performed using a machine with a pulley system. Although people feel they must stand straight up when they do it, it's actually better to be slightly flexed forward at the waist, with your back slightly arched. When you stand straight up, you're asking your abdominal muscles to support your torso so you can perform the exercise. Eventually, your triceps will become so strong that you'll begin placing too much stress on the abdominal muscles to support the torso during the exercise. By bending forward slightly, your hip flexors and quadriceps kick in to help support the position. Bend your knees slightly, keeping your knees over your feet, and weight bear mostly through your heels. Your shoulders, knees, and feet should all remain in vertical alignment throughout the exercise.

To start, grip the bar with your hands shoulder width apart near your chest. Keep your elbows against your body throughout the motion; don't let them rise. Slowly lower the bar until your hands

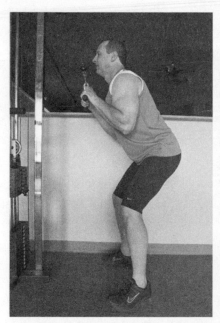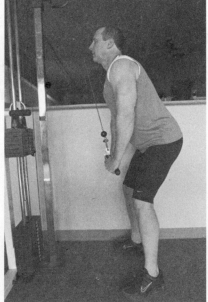

FIGURE 5.49 Triceps extension. The start, left, and the finish, right.

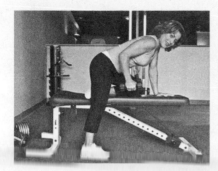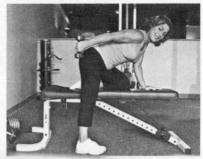

FIGURE 5.50 Kick-backs. The start, left, and the finish, right.

touch your thighs, but don't lock your elbows. Slowly return the weights to the start position near your chest, making sure you go through the full range of motion, chest to thighs. Stand close enough to the pulley so when you pull the cable, it comes almost straight down.

Kick-backs: This is an optional triceps exercise requiring only dumbbells, so you can perform it if no other devices are available. Place one knee on a bench and place your same side hand on the bench, in line with your knee. Place the opposite foot slightly wider than shoulder width away from the bench and slightly behind the knee on the bench. Point the foot on the floor forward and bend the knee slightly. Grip a dumbbell in your free arm, and start with your forearm perpendicular to the floor and your palm facing your body. Bring your forearm back until it's just below parallel to the floor and just before you lock your elbow. Return it to the start position. Throughout the exercise, make sure your upper arm remains just below parallel to the floor and your forearm runs right along your body and doesn't flare out.

6

STRETCH, DON'T STRAIN

Stretching is an important part of the initial stage of an exercise program. As you've already learned, for every muscle, there's an opposing muscle that pulls the other way. If one of these muscles becomes stronger than the opposing muscle, an imbalance forms. Through the course of the day, all your muscles move to some degree. Blood flows through them to keep them warm and flexible. While you sleep, muscles shorten from lack of movement. If there's an imbalance, the stronger muscle shortens, because the other muscle isn't strong enough to offset the contractility of this muscle. As a result, you wake with tight muscles. Many of my therapy patients say they feel great after they stretch in the morning, but by the next morning they're tight again. Now you understand why. Stretching is only a short-term solution. Correcting a muscle imbalance is the key to sustaining muscle length and good flexibility.

Maintaining proper muscle length is important because a muscle creates its greatest force at its normal length. If it's shortened or lengthened too much, it loses its ability to create force. A shortened

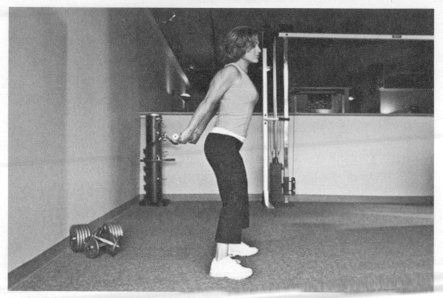

FIGURE 6.1 Improper shoulder stretch.

muscle also is susceptible to strain if overstretched quickly during a functional activity. Anyone who's strained (pulled) a hamstring muscle while running to first base or reaching for a ball on the tennis court can attest to this.

As valuable as stretching is, it's possible to overstretch, and this can cause more harm than good. I've seen people attempt to stretch his or her shoulders by holding a wand behind their back and rotating their arms so the wand touches their lower back. By doing this, they're overstretching the ligaments of the front of their shoulders, creating a level of instability (see Figure 6.1). Gymnasts, for instance, become so flexible that their spines become unstable, because they've stretched out the muscles of the spine and the ligaments surrounding the spine. This often leads to back problems and hip injuries later in life. To be flexible, you need only move a joint within a normal range and not beyond.

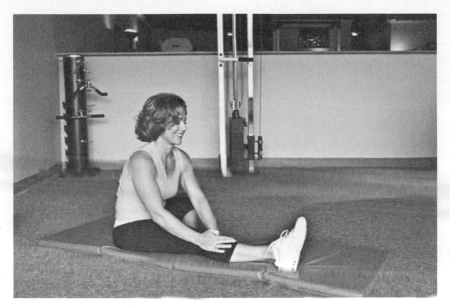

FIGURE 6.2 Hamstring stretch.

The Legs

Let's continue with the legs. Tightness in the lower-extremity musculature is common, because these muscles work hard during the course of the day. If a muscle imbalance exists in the legs, it will be exaggerated.

Hamstring Stretch: Extend the leg you are stretching out in front of you. If you're doing this on a table, hang your other leg over the side. Otherwise, bend your knee and place your foot near the knee of the leg being stretched. Start with your back straight and upright and slowly lean forward until you feel a mild stretch in your hamstrings (group of muscles at the back of the thigh). Remember to keep your back straight or mildly arched, but not hunched. If you hunch, you're stretching your lower back and not your hamstrings. The knee of the stretched leg should remain fully extended. Some

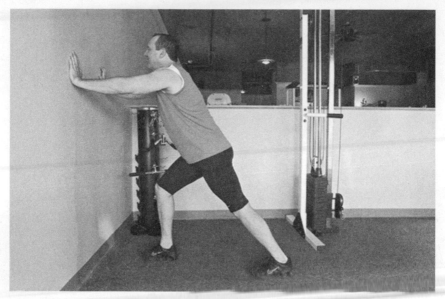

FIGURE 6.3 Calf stretch.

people might not be able to attain a full upright position. In this case, just come as close to an upright position as you can. Then, place your hand behind you on the table to support yourself while you're stretching. Your goal is to bring your chest toward the leg being stretched while never giving up the straight or mildly arched back position.

Calf Stretch: The most common way to stretch the calf is to stand facing a wall and extend the leg of the calf you're stretching behind you. Keep the knee of this leg straight, and bend the other knee slightly. With your hands on the wall, slowly lean forward, without allowing your back heel to come off the floor. Hold the stretch for thirty seconds, then alternate legs.

Quadriceps Stretch: For this stretch, you'll need a sturdy object behind you to place your foot on and something in front of you for support and balance. Two chairs work well. Place the foot of the

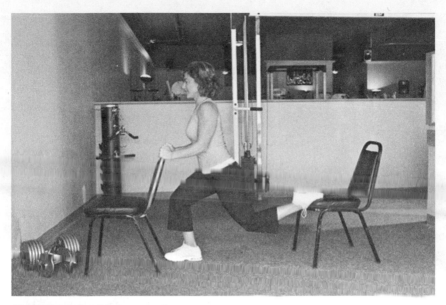

FIGURE 6.4 Quadriceps stretch.

leg you're stretching on the chair seat behind you. Place the other chair far enough in front of you for the knee of the stretching leg to be behind your hip. Start to sit back as if you were going to sit on your back foot. Continue until you feel the stretch. Keep your front knee over your front foot, not in front of it, and your back slightly hunched for the best stretch possible. Don't be surprised if you can't actually sit on the heel of the back leg. The quadriceps passes the hip and knee, so if you start the stretch with your knee behind your hip, you're already stretching the quadriceps. As you sit back and bend at the knee, you're continuing the stretch. Because not all the stretch is occurring at the knee, your butt won't reach your heel. Most people only stretch at the knee. Unless you stretch at the hip and knee as described, you're not getting a complete stretch.

Adductor Stretch: The inner thigh, or groin, is a common area for sports-related injuries. To stretch this area, sit on the floor with

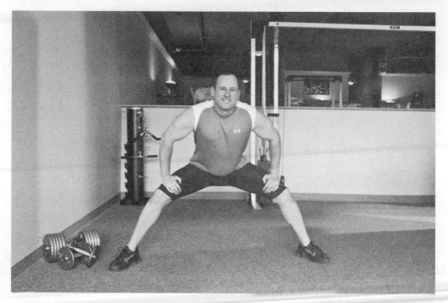

FIGURE 6.5 Adductor stretch

knees bent and feet touching each other sole to sole, with the outsides of your feet on the floor. Place your forearms on your inner thighs and grab your ankles. Slowly press your thighs down to the floor with your forearms. To stretch the part of the adductor that passes the knee (the *gracilis*), stand up and spread your feet apart as far as you can, keeping your toes facing forward. You can place your hands on your thighs to help maintain your balance. Unlike the sitting stretch, where you feel the pull of the muscle toward your groin, in this stretch you'll feel the pull of the muscle more toward your knee. This is because when you keep your knee straight, it forces you to stretch the one muscle of the adductor group that passes the knee and, as a result, you feel the stretch closer to the knee.

Abductor Stretch: The abductor muscle region is the hip, also known as the lateral portion of the pelvis. These muscles are re-

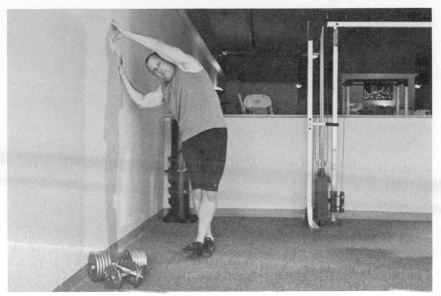

FIGURE 6.6 Abductor stretch.

sponsible for maintaining balance when one foot is off the floor and when you're standing on just one leg, such as when walking. They also work in conjunction with the lower back muscles to help stabilize the torso and pelvis so your arm and leg muscles have a stable point to pull off of. It's not uncommon for these muscles to become tight, so maintaining them at their proper length through stretching is important.

This stretch is the opposite of the groin stretch. Hold onto the side of a doorway with your feet close to the doorway. Place the foot of the leg you'll be stretching—let's say it's the left leg—in front of and across the right foot. Place your right hand just above head height on the doorway, and place your left hand at waist height on the doorway. Slowly begin to move the left hip out to the side. You'll be bending your torso to make a "C" shape with your hip at the apex of the C. Wait until you feel a comfortable stretch, then hold it for thirty seconds.

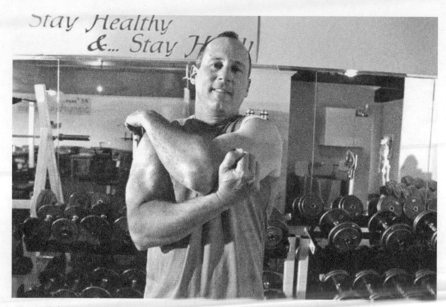

FIGURE 6.7 Shoulder region stretch

Shoulder Region Stretch: To stretch between the shoulder blades, grab the arm to be stretched by the triceps region (just above the elbow) and pull it across, in front of your body until you feel a stretch between your shoulder blades. Hold it for thirty seconds. To stretch the front of the shoulders, clasp your hands behind your back and pull them up and away from your body until you feel the stretch. To stretch the triceps and posterior region of the shoulders, grab the triceps region with the other hand over your head and the elbow bent. Push the elbow back.

Pecs Stretch: Standing in a doorway, raise your elbows to just below shoulder height and place them on either side of the doorjamb. If your elbows don't reach, hold the doorjamb with your hands, keeping your elbows just below shoulder height. Slowly lean into the doorway until you feel a stretch at the pecs (chest). Hold for thirty seconds.

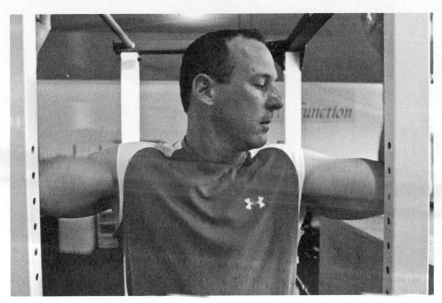

FIGURE 6.8 Pecs stretch.

7

A WORKOUT SCHEDULE
THAT WORKS FOR YOU

This book is designed to be used in two distinct fashions: first, as a mechanism for resolving pain that can be attributed to muscle weakness; second, as a means of developing a weight-training program to maximize the function of the muscular system and prevent injuries.

If you are using the book to resolve pain as the result of muscle weakness, setting up a workout program is easy. Simply use the exercises designated for each cause as described in Chapter 3. Perform the groups of exercises two or three times a week. If your schedule does not allow you to perform the routines three times a week, don't be concerned. Exercising the specific muscles noted twice a week will get the job done. What is important is that the technique for each exercise performed is good and the resistance utilized is correct.

If you are using the book to set up a workout program for general conditioning, two methods fit most people's needs. If you can work out only a couple of times a week for short periods of time, the weight-training progress chart outlines the exercise that is most important for each body part. This method is also good for individuals just starting out weight lifting and for people concerned about becoming overwhelmed by the number of exercises suggested to complete a full workout routine.

If would like to complete a full routine, the weight-training progress chart indicates many exercises for each body part. The chart provides suggestions for alternatives depending on equipment requirements as well as optional exercises for further isolation of muscles or parts of muscle groups. The weight-training progress chart, when followed correctly, will allow an individual to perform no more than three or four exercises for any body part.

Once you determine how much time you can devote to weight training, the next question is how to break up the exercises into a complete workout. If you choose to perform the abridged workout routine (one exercise per body part), the same exercises will be performed during each workout. I suggest that no body part be worked out more than twice a week, and in most cases once a week is sufficient. Don't forget, it is the amount of weight you use for an exercise that ultimately causes the muscle to grow and get stronger, not how many times you perform the exercise. In this case, you will perform the same workout routine just twice a week. That is all that is necessary to achieve a workout routine that will maintain good strength of all muscles and will produce increased strength gains but at a slower rate than the more complete workout routine.

If you choose to perform the complete workout routine, this can be achieved by working out either two or three times per week. There are six main muscle groups; legs, chest, back, shoulders, biceps, and triceps. If you choose to work out twice a week, you'll work three body parts each session; at three times a week, you'll work two body parts per session. To decide which muscles to work in a session, look at the size of the muscles in the separate groups and distribute them accordingly. Your legs are the biggest group in size, so a good setup for the two-day system would be to group leg exercises with the smaller muscles of the shoulders and biceps in one session, and chest, back, and triceps into another. For the three-day system, work your legs and shoulders one day, your back and triceps another day, and your chest and biceps on a third day. You can work your abs during each session, whether you choose two sessions a week or three. The important thing is to take at least one day in between workouts to allow the muscles to heal and grow. You should be able to complete each workout in ninety minutes on the two-day system and in sixty minutes on the three-day system.

Your energy level is the other consideration in determining your workout routine. If you find it difficult to sustain enough energy to get good results through a ninety-minute, two-day routine, don't just go through the motions; switch to the three-day routine. You want to get the most out of each workout. If you can spare only thirty to forty-five minutes a day, I recommend performing the abridged workout routine twice a week.

Regardless of which schedule you choose, the important thing to remember is that muscle grows one or two days after a workout. Therefore, you don't want to work the same muscle group any quicker than three days apart. This includes aerobic exercise. If you work your legs on a particular day, I wouldn't recommend even aerobic exercise for the next day or two, to allow your muscles to grow, unimpeded. Muscles heal during your off days, and this takes energy. If you try to work out on a day when your body is healing, you may not have enough energy to perform your exercise and you may cause the muscles to strain because they are in the healing phase and are not prepared to be stressed by exercise.

As mentioned earlier, complete physical fitness requires strength, flexibility, and stamina. Unfortunately, most people don't have time in their schedules for both weight training and aerobic exercise. If you have time in the week to perform only one type of exercise, I unequivocally recommend weight training over any form of cardiovascular exercise such as running or cycling. Weight training can raise the resting metabolic rate like no other form of exercise, so it's the best exercise for losing weight or, more specifically, for making the body use fat more effectively. Strength training is just as effective at improving the function of the cardiovascular system as aerobic exercise. Strength training also simulates functional activities much more closely than aerobic exercise. Most functional activities, including most sports, are performed over short durations at high intensities, not at comfortable speeds for thirty minutes to an hour. Performing the average strength-training set takes no more than ten seconds. After you've completed your weight training, if you want to perform aerobic exercise, go ahead. But if you have to choose between the two, choose weight training.

Regardless of how you break it down, an effective full-body workout schedule shouldn't require much more than a three-hour-a-week commitment. If you can't find three hours a week for yourself, you're not looking hard enough!

Conclusion

Weight training has had a profound impact on my life. The change in my physique has made me feel so much better about myself that my confidence has skyrocketed. Putting fifty pounds of muscle on when the predisposition of my body was to be thin made me realize there was nothing I couldn't accomplish as long as I put my mind and heart into it. The fear of failure, which stops so many people from living their dreams, was erased forever in me, and I began to establish other major goals for my life. When I decided on physical therapy as my career, it seemed like divine intervention. I was now going to help people overcome obstacles and get them back to the lives they had lost. It's ironic that a former ninety-nine-pound weakling is now teaching and representing to people that getting stronger can resolve pain and allow for normal function.

My feelings about what I've accomplished are never far from my mind. That's why I find it so easy to empathize with my patients and personal-training clients. These people are looking to me to resolve their issues—whether it's life-altering pain, a poor physique, or a weight issue that is affecting someone's health or self-esteem. I know from experience that these problems don't have quick solutions. To resolve them takes time and effort. My job is to educate both my patients and my personal-training clients on what they need to do to help themselves and also to motivate them to accomplish their goals. I've found that, in most cases, the ability to heal lies within the injured individual. I think of my patients and my clients as my children. A client is like a child who wants to ride a bike but doesn't know how. I'm not going to ride the bike for the client. I'm going to teach him what to do and then cheer him on. I have to sit back and see if he takes my information and uses it to ride the bike. In strength training, keeping the body in good shape is the task.

What concerns me is that the medical community sometimes fails people. In most of the cases I have treated, turning to a physician for information about pain resolution is futile. The diagnosis and treatment often appear to be one-sided. Often, the only method used to determine the cause of pain is through diagnostic tests such as x-rays or MRIs. These show only structural abnormalities that may have nothing to do with the cause of one's pain. In my fifteen years of experience treating patients, I've found that, in close to 80 percent, the cause of pain has been muscular. Treatment protocols, including medication and surgeries, are performed because the true cause is never established. I have prevented a substantial number of patients from receiving unnecessary surgery because I was able to resolve their symptoms through strength training.

I want to help you make better, more informed decisions about your health, to decipher whether your symptoms can be resolved through strength training or whether they require medical attention. The medical community's knee-jerk reaction to take an x-ray or an MRI to diagnose the cause of pain eliminates the possibility that the cause of a symptom may be in another location. The body works like a big chain. Sometimes, one link breaks because another has weakened and has placed too much stress on that link. I've treated a number of patients whose ankle pains were the result of weak hip muscles, which caused them to weight bear improperly through the ankle, causing the ankle muscles to break down.

Strengthening hip muscles resolved the ankle pain. You have to evaluate the body as a whole to come up with the correct cause of symptoms. Anti-inflammatories, muscle relaxants, painkillers, and cortisone shots won't solve the problem.

I realize I'm bucking the medical establishment when I say that most pain experienced on a daily basis that limits function is caused by muscular deficits and not by structural ones such as herniated discs, arthritis, or vertebral subluxations. There is nothing malicious about this; I'm merely pointing out a flaw in the way the medical community has been trained. Most physicians don't understand the way muscles contribute to the cause of pain because those responsible for treating pain are either orthopedic surgeons trained to reconstruct the skeletal system or neurologists and chiropractors trained to correct nerve-related problems. Muscle problems don't fit into their educational or training background. I've seen this firsthand through treating patients after they were diagnosed with structural deficits. Some came to me because the physician thought physical therapy was advisable, but in most cases, the patients came to me because they were referred by former patients of mine. If the cause of a symptom was structural, I would refer the patient to the proper specialist for treatment. But if I thought the cause was muscular, I would have the patient begin a strength-building regimen.

I want to take what I've been able to accomplish at my office to a larger audience. I hope you're willing to try. I changed my life through strength training; allow me the opportunity to help change yours.

Acknowledgments

I would like to thank Bob Nadelman for assisting me in the development of this book. He became a true believer in aggressive strength training as the means to resolving pain after he was told by his doctor that his pain was the result of a lower back nerve root problem that would require surgery. He found me through his racquetball partner, and I proved the pain was actually a muscle in spasm and the symptoms down his legs were the result of the muscle impinging on his sciatic nerve. Within six weeks of starting therapy he was back to playing racquetball. As a result of this revelation, he felt that my already completed strength training book could be more valuable if I added a chapter describing how I am able to determine whether pain is the result of a structural or muscular problem. I completed the chapter, and changed the book's title to Overpower Pain.

Thank you to Nancy Feldman for editing the book. Most people who have read anything I have written state that it sounds just like the way I talk. Nancy took the time and the effort to clean up the text and make it concise and proper. My ideas were retained but greatly improved through Nancy's efforts. I enjoyed working with Nancy because she wanted me to make sure that the ideas were described in a way that any lay person could understand them.

Finally, I would like to thank Judy Aaron for being a good friend during all my trials and tribulations. I met Judy before I even opened PT2. We hit it off and I told her she would be working at my office once it opened. That was over twelve years ago. She has seen me develop my ideas and change from a local physical therapist to a man trying to change the way pain causation and resolution is perceived. She has been very supportive and willing to listen to all the dreams and ideas that float around in my brain. She has never been shy about giving me her opinion about the things I intended to do. Over time, I have come to the conclusion that there are very few people in life that you can trust to be there when you need them. Judy has always been one of them, and I feel she deserves recognition for that.

Glossary

A

Achilles tendon: The tendon that attaches the muscles of the back of the shin or the calf to the heel bone.

abdominal sheath: The wall of the abdominal cavity that incorporates the muscles of this region. They include the rectus abdominis, the internal and external obliques, and the transversus abdominis.

abductor: A muscle that draws a body part away from the body.

acromium process: A flattened portion of bone that juts out over the shoulder joint to prevent the upper arm bone from moving upward and out of the shoulder joint when the arm is raised up or to the side.

actin: One of two proteins that make up muscle tissue. A muscle contraction occurs when actin comes in contact with the other protein, myosin.

active range of motion: The measured range of motion that an individual can achieve at a joint without assistance.

adductor: A muscle that draws a body part in toward the body.

aerobic: "With oxygen." An exercise performed in a state during which the body's oxygen requirement is being met.

anaerobic: "Without oxygen." An exercise performed without sufficient oxygen. An exercising individual would find it difficult to breathe when performing an activity anaerobically, and lactic acid would develop in this environment.

anterior cruciate ligament (ACL): One of two ligaments that attach from the femur to the tibia in the knee joint. (The other is the posterior cruciate ligament.) These ligaments are responsible for preventing the tibia from sliding too far forward or backward in relation to the femur. In addition, they prevent too much rotation and hyperextension/hyperflexion at the knee joint.

anterior tibialis: A muscle at the front of the shin that passes the ankle and attaches to a couple of ankle bones. It's responsible for bending the ankle so the foot flexes (moves toward the face).

anterior tilt: An improper position (posture) of the pelvis, in which the front or anterior portion has moved downward toward the floor. It is typically the result of a muscle-strength imbalance between the quadriceps (front thigh) muscles and the hamstrings (posterior thigh) muscles.

B

barbell: A piece of equipment used in weight lifting that consists of a steel bar with weights on both ends. The weights are secured by collars, to prevent them from sliding off.

benign: An abnormality of the structure of a tissue that is not threatening to one's life or health.

biceps: The muscle found at the front of the upper arm that attaches from the elbow to the shoulder. Its primary function is to bend the elbow, but it can also help to lift an arm held in front, from the shoulder.

biceps tuberosity: A small protuberance at the end of the radius bone, where the tendon of the biceps muscle attaches.

binding sites: The points where contact is made between the two proteins of muscle fiber, actin, and myosin.

biomechanics: The study of the way joints, bones, and muscles move and the forces that create these movements.

bone density: The amount of bone minerals present in a given area of bone. As bone is lost, a pathology known as osteopenia develops. As the density decreases further, a pathology known as osteoporosis develops.

bone spur: A small calcium deposit or an outpouching from existing bone.

brachialis: A muscle that attaches from the upper portion of the upper arm bone (humerus), passes the elbow joint, and attaches to the ulna, in the forearm.

brachioradialis: A muscle that attaches from the lower portion of the humerus to the farthest, most distal portion of the radius. The attachment to the radius is near the wrist.

bulging disc: A disc in which the nucleus pulposus has shifted from the center of a disc but is still inside the line of the vertebral column.

bursa: A purse of fluid that sits between two tissues to reduce friction and pain.

bursitis: Inflammation and pain around a bursa.

C

cardiovascular system: The heart and circulatory vessels (arteries and veins), responsible for transporting blood to all the cells of the body.

carpal tunnel syndrome: An altered sensation consisting of pain, numbness, burning, or tingling in the thumb, index finger, middle finger, and half the ring finger. Carpal tunnel syndrome results from compression of the median nerve that travels across the carpal tunnel (bottom of the wrist). The nerve becomes impinged on by the tendons that lead to the wrist and fingers that flex them.

cerebrospinal fluid: Found in the cavities within the brain and around the surface of the brain and the spinal cord. This fluid provides nutrients to the spinal cord and discs. It also controls pressure around the brain and spinal cord.

chondromalacia patellae: Softening of the cartilage at the back, or underside, of the kneecap. It's also referred to as patellofemoral syndrome (PFS). The cartilage covering the bone, which is the surface of the kneecap that glides through the knee joint, can soften and become inflamed, creating pain at the back of the kneecap.

contractile force: The amount of force a muscle creates as it contracts. This force even exists when a muscle is at rest—a state known as resting tone.

contusion: A type of injury without laceration, resulting from an impact; a bruise.

coracoid process: A portion of bone at the shoulder blade that helps form the inner boundary of the shoulder joint.

D

diabetes mellitus: A disease caused by an insulin deficiency and characterized by an excess of sugar in the blood and urine.

disc: The material between the vertebrae (bones of the spine). The disc is comprised of a gel-like substance surrounded by dense cartilage. The gel has the ability to accept shock and help support the spine; the cartilage keeps the gel in the center of the disc.

dorsiflexor: A muscle that passes the ankle joint and causes the ankle to move up toward the face.

dumbbell: A weight held in one hand for the purpose of weight lifting. Dumbbells can come in preset weights or a single bar that individual weights can be loaded onto.

E

electrical stimulation: The use of a small current of electricity to achieve an altered physiological effect such as decreased pain or swelling or increased strength of a muscle.

electromyography (EMG): A diagnostic test used to determine whether sensory and motor nerves are functioning properly.

erector spinae: A muscle group of the lower back region that attaches to various portions of the spine. Along with the quadratus lumborum, it is responsible for stability of the back region.

evertor: A muscle of the ankle that bends the ankle out.

F

femur: The thighbone. This is the longest and strongest bone in the body.

G

gastrocnemius: The largest calf muscle. It attaches to the ankle via the Achilles tendon, passes the knee joint, and attaches to the bottom of the femur (thighbone). The gastrocnemius flexes the ankle downward and can help flex or bend the knee.

glenoid fossa (glenoid cavity): The concave end of the shoulder blade or scapula, which receives the upper portion of the humerus to form the shoulder joint.

gluteal muscles (glutes): The muscles found in the buttocks region. They include the gluteus maximus, gluteus medius, and gluteus minimus.

gracilis: The portion of the adductor muscle that passes the knee.

H

hamstrings: Group of posterior thigh muscles. They pass on both sides of the knee as they reach their attachment points on the tibia and the fibula (lower leg bones). They are responsible for flexing and bending the knee. They also perform hip extension.

herniated disc: When a disc's gel-like inner portion partially shifts outside the line of the vertebral column but is still encapsulated by the outer portion.

humerus: Upper arm bone.

hyaline cartilage: The layer of cartilage found on joint surfaces. Its glasslike surface allows movement of a joint without jeopardizing the end of a bone.

hyperextend: Forcing a joint beyond its normal range of motion. This can strain the joint capsule and ligaments that provide stability at the end range of motion of a joint.

I

iliac crest: The top rim of the back of the pelvis.

iliotibial band (ITB): A long band of connective tissue that attaches from the pelvis to the knee. Because the band passes by the hip, it can move the leg to the side, which is known as abducting.

immune system: The white blood cells, spleen, and other tissues that are responsible for recognizing and eliminating foreign organisms or substances in the body.

inflammatory response: The body's protective response to illness or injury, characterized by pain, redness, heat, and dysfunction.

infraspinatus: See **supraspinatus**

intercondylar groove: At the end of the femur (thighbone) are two rounded elements called condyles. Between them is a space (a depression) called the intercondylar groove (or intercondylar fossa), where the kneecap is situated. As the knee is straightened or bent, the kneecap glides through this groove.

invertor: A muscle that causes an inward turning movement of a part of the body such as the ankle. The ankle's invertor also helps support the arch of the foot to prevent flatfootedness.

L

lactic acid: A byproduct of muscular contraction. Each time a muscle contracts, lactic acid develops. Lactic acid can prevent a muscle from contracting by limiting the two proteins that make up muscle from binding together. Once a muscle stops contracting, the circulatory system removes lactic acid from a muscle and brings it to the liver to be processed and converted into pyruvic acid, which can then be used for energy, if needed.

latissimus dorsi (lats): Two broad, triangular muscles that lie flat across the back. They attach from the upper portion of the arm on both sides, all the way down to the top of the pelvis and medially to a large portion of the spine.

length-tension ratio: The relationship between the length of a muscle and its ability to create force. A muscle at either a shortened length or an extended length loses its ability to create force, and a muscle at the midrange creates the greatest force.

ligamentous tissue: The ligaments (or connective tissue) that attach one bone to another at a joint. It could also include the joint capsule, because in many joints, the ligaments fuse with the joint capsule, which surrounds the joint and is composed of the same connective tissue as the ligaments.

lower trapezius: Draws the shoulder blade down toward the floor at the end range of shoulder flexion (with the arm raised from shoulder height to overhead).

M

massage: The use of hand movements over an area of the body to facilitate an altered physiological state such as decreased swelling, decreased pain, decreased knotting in a muscle, or increased circulation.

mass building: Weight lifting performed to increase muscle mass.

mechanical deficit: Situation in which there is nothing structurally wrong with the tissue in question except that a muscle or muscles are applying an improper force on the tissue, causing pain.

median nerve: The nerve that emanates from several nerve roots of the cervical (neck) spinal cord. The median nerve travels down the arm and ends in the fingers and provides both sensory (touch) aspects to the skin and motor contraction to the muscles in the forearm and hand.

meniscal cartilage (meniscus): Fibrous connective tissue cushion that sits at the knee joint between the femur and the tibia. It is broken up into two parts: the inner half (medial meniscus) and the outer half (lateral meniscus). It provides shock absorption to the knee joint when standing or moving and helps direct an individual's body weight to the ground.

meniscal tear: A tear of the meniscal cartilage that can occur if the knee is overstretched (extended), overbent (flexed), or severely twisted while the foot is planted on the ground.

metabolic rate: The rate at which the body burns calories to perform essential functions such as circulation, digestion, and respiration. This rate can change, based on the amount and type of tissue the body must maintain.

metabolism: The system of chemical activities that maintain life by fueling the body's processes, activities, and growth.

microtear: Tiny tear in the muscles that occurs during weight lifting, which cause the weight lifter to feel sore a day or two after lifting. The body's response to these minor tears is to produce more muscle. These tears do not reduce a muscle's ability to create force.

middle trapezius (mid-trap): A portion of the trapezius muscle that attaches from the skull to the thoracic portion of the spine. The mid-trap portion attaches from the medial portion of the shoulder blades to the spine and covers the rhomboids.

momentum: A force created when you put a joint through its range of motion quickly. If you lift quickly, you're using momentum rather than muscle, thus receiving no strength-training benefit from the exercise.

muscle groups: Groups of muscles that work together to perform a movement or action.

muscle mass: The overall amount of muscle tissue present in an individual's body.

myosin: See **actin**

N

negatives: The stage of an exercise where the muscle is lengthening. For a muscle to go through full motion, it must first shorten to the farthest point permitted by the joint it is passing. It then returns to the starting point by lengthening back to its full length. The lengthening stage is called the eccentric contraction or negative portion.

O

obliques: Located on the sides of the abdominal region, a muscle group that includes the internal and external obliques. They attach from the ribs to the sides of the rectus abdominis muscle. The obliques and the rectus abdominis create the abdominal wall.

orthotic: A device placed in the shoe to assist in creating mechanical assistance to the foot. These devices are designed to resolve pain at the foot by providing an external support (force) to the foot.

osteoarthritis: A degeneration of cartilage and its underlying bone within a joint, causing inflammation and often causing pain.

osteoporosis: A disease in which bone density and mass are lost, causing sufferers to become more susceptible to fractures.

P

passive range of motion: The measured amount of motion that can be achieved by another person moving an individual's joint without the individual's assistance.

physical therapist: A licensed health provider who uses different forms of treatment such as hot packs, cold packs, electric stimulation, ultrasound, massage, and other modalities, weight lifting and other exercises and training to correct symptoms such as pain or reduced range of motion at a joint, to allow an individual to return to normal function.

piriformis: A muscle found in the buttocks or gluteal region that runs from the sacral spine to the hip joint. It is located very close to the sciatic nerve, and in some people, the sciatic nerve passes through the muscle as the nerve starts its way down the leg.

plantar fascia: A broad, flat band of connective tissue that attaches from the five balls of the feet (metatarsal heads) to the heel (calcaneus). The tissue helps to support the arch of the foot. When inflamed or overstretched, the plantar fascia will display pain either along the underside of the foot or just at the plantar fascia's attachment at the heel.

plantar flexor: A muscle that passes the ankle joint and causes the ankle to move away from the face.

posterior deltoid (post-delts): The portion of the deltoid at the back of the shoulder. The posterior deltoid attaches from the shoulder blade to the upper arm.

progressive resistance weight training: The use of progressively increasing resistance with weight-training exercises to cause a muscle to respond by increasing muscle mass, allowing the muscle to develop more strength.

pulmonary system: The organs from the nose to the lungs responsible for the intake of oxygen from the air and the removal of carbon dioxide from the body.

pyruvic acid: The final byproduct of the breakdown of glucose.

Q

quadratus lumborum: Muscles of the lower back region. They are responsible for stability in the back region and attach from the ribs to the top of the pelvis.

quadriceps (quads): Front thigh muscles. Four muscle bellies make up the quads, which attach to the kneecap and control its position in the knee joint. The quadriceps are responsible for extending and straightening the knee.

R

radius: One of the two bones of the forearm.

rectus abdominis: The muscle at the front of the abdominal region. Because this muscle attaches from the rib cage to the front of the pelvis, as it contracts, it brings these two regions together, creating the motion of hunching. The muscle's main function is to help support and protect the organs in the abdominal region, such as the large and small intestines.

referred pain: Pain felt in one area that is created by inflammation of a tissue in another area. An example is pain in the left arm when someone is having a heart attack. Referred symptoms can result from inflammation of muscles, nerves, bones, or organs.

repetition (rep): The completion of the movement being performed in an exercise. A rep is usually both repeated and counted.

resistance: The force that a muscle works against to cause the muscle to adapt by building muscle tissue. This force can be created with dumbbells, weight stacks on machines, cuff weights, or resistance bands.

retinaculum: A structure consisting of connective tissue that holds an organ or tissue in place.

rhomboids: A group of muscles that assist in stabilizing the shoulder blades. The rhomboids attach horizontally between the shoulder blades and to the upper spine.

rotator cuff: A group of four muscles, the subscapularis, supraspinatus, infraspinatus, and teres minor, that acts to surround and support the head of the humerus (upper arm bone) and keep it in the shoulder joint.

S

sciatica: Pain, burning, or tingling from the gluteal region or buttocks, down the side or back of the leg to the foot. Most doctors contend that the cause of sciatica is a herniated disc pinching on a nerve root. The author maintains that sciatica is the result of a strained muscle, the piriformis, in the buttocks region. The strain causes swelling, which pinches the sciatic nerve, causing the described symptoms.

sciatic nerve: A nerve comprised of seven nerve roots from the lumbar and sacral (section of the spine below the lower back region that attaches to the pelvis) regions of the spine. The sciatic nerve provides nerve impulses to many of the muscles of the leg and provides sensation to the lower leg and foot below the knee.

set: A group of repetitions of an exercise.

shin splints: A common name for anterior tibialis tendonitis, shin splints is a syndrome where pain is felt at the front of the shin. This can result either from a strain of the anterior tibialis or irritation of the connective tissue covering the tibia, which is the shin bone that the anterior tibialis connects to.

shocking the muscle: The act of changing, on a regular basis, the exercises or the sequence of exercises performed in your routine.

soleus: The portion of the calf muscle that attaches to the two bones of the lower leg (the tibia and fibula). This muscle is responsible strictly for bending the ankle so the toes point away from the face.

spasm: An involuntary continuous contraction of a muscle. It is typically caused by a muscle being shortened excessively, strained, or contracted for an extended period of time.

stenosis: Shrinkage or narrowing of a joint space, blood vessel or organ.

strength training: See **weight training**

structural deficit: Situation in which the presence of pain is caused by something implicitly wrong with the tissue, which is preventing the tissue from properly performing its function.

subacromial bursa: A bursa that sits between the acromium process and the head of the humerus to prevent friction between the tendons that pass through this subacromial space and the acromium process.

supersetting: Performing two sets of exercises back-to-back with no rest. This could mean performing the same exercise with different weights or performing different exercises.

supraspinatus: One of the four muscles that comprise the rotator cuff. The supraspinatus attaches above and below the spine of the scapula (a protrusion on the back of the shoulder blade that separates the supraspinatus from the infraspinatus, another of the four muscles of the rotator cuff).

T

tendonitis: Inflammation of a tendon

tensor fascia lata: A small muscle that's attached to the iliotibial band (ITB). Because the ITB is made of connective tissue and can't move or create force, the tensor fascia lata, which sits atop the ITB near the hip, acts upon the ITB to allow it to move the leg out to the side.

teres major: Muscle that works in conjunction with the latissimus dorsi to move the arm. The teres major is attached from the upper portion of the arm to the lateral portion of the shoulder blade.

thoracolumbar fascia: The connective tissue that attaches the latissimus dorsi to the pelvis and lumbar spine.

tibia: Lower leg bone. The tibia sits below the femur (the thighbone) and combines with the femur to make up the knee joint. It's the main weight-bearing bone of the lower leg.

toning: Weight training performed to teach a muscle to be more effective in its ability to utilize lactic acid and in its ability to sustain muscle contractions for longer periods of time.

torque: Rotational force. The force is defined by the amount of resistance or weight used to perform an exercise, multiplied by the distance from the pivot point or the joint where the force is being created.

trapezius: A muscle that attaches from the skull to the shoulder blades and along the spine down to the mid back. It is usually described in three parts: the upper trapezius, the middle trapezius, and the lower trapezius.

triceps: The muscle at the back of the upper arm. The triceps attaches at the back of the elbow and at the shoulder and is responsible for extending (straightening) the elbow. It can also help to pull the arm backward from the shoulder.

trochanteric bursa: Bursa that sits between the ITB and the head of the femur as it enters the hip joint. The purpose of the trochanteric bursa is to prevent inflammation of these tissues as they move across one another during hip movement.

U

ultrasound: The therapeutic or diagnostic use of high-frequency sound waves directed over an area of the body. Ultrasound can be used in therapy to create an altered physiological state such as increased circulation, decreased pain, or decreased scar tissue development.

upper trapezius: Upper back muscle that helps to elevate the shoulders and support the head.

V

venous flow: The speed at which blood flows through veins as it returns from tissues back to the heart.

vertebral subluxation: A condition where one or more bones of the spine move out of position and irritate the spinal nerves.

W

weight lifting: The use of any device—including dumbbells, barbells, machines, resistance tubes, or band—that provides resistance and increases muscle strength with proper use.

weight training (or strength training): The lifting of weights, performed on a regular schedule to improve or maintain muscle strength.

APPENDIX A: WEIGHT-TRAINING PROGRESS CHART

DATE →						
	QUADS	WT/REPS	WT/REPS	WT/REPS	WT/REPS	WT/REPS
Primary	*Squats set 1					
	2					
	3					
	OR (choose one)					
	Lunges set 1					
	2					
	3					
Secondary	Knee extensions set 1					
	2					
	3					
	OR (choose one)					
	Leg Press 1					
	2					
	3					
	HAMSTRINGS					
Primary	*Straight Leg Deadlifts 1					
	2					
	3					
Secondary	Hamstring Curl 1					
	2					
	3					
	HIPS					
Primary	Hip Abduction 1					
	2					
	3					
Optional	Hip Adduction 1					
	2					
	3					

*Asterisk marks key exercise for this body part. If you perform only one exercise for this body part, do this one.

APPENDIX A: WEIGHT-TRAINING PROGRESS CHART						
DATE →						
	LOWER LEG	WT/REPS	WT/REPS	WT/REPS	WT/REPS	WT/REPS
Primary	*Donkey Calf 1 2 3					
Secondary	Seated Calf 1 2 3					
Secondary	Toe Raise 1 2 3					
	CHEST					
Primary	*Flat Bench Press 1 2 3					
Secondary	Flyes 1 2 3					
Secondary	Incline Bench Press 1 2 3					
	BACK					
Primary	T-Bar Rows 1 2 3 *OR Barbell Rows 1 2 3 *OR One-Arm Rows 1 2					

APPENDIX A: WEIGHT-TRAINING PROGRESS CHART

	DATE →					
	BACK (cont.)	WT/REPS	WT/REPS	WT/REPS	WT/REPS	WT/REPS
Secondary	*Seated Pulley Row 1 2 3					
Secondary	Lat Pulldown Behind Neck 1 2 3					
Secondary	Lat Pulldown with Neutral Bar 1 2 3					
Optional	Hyperextensions 1 2 3					
	SHOULDERS					
Primary	*Seated Military Press 1 2 3					
Optional	Front Laterals 1 2 3					
Optional	Side Laterals 1 2 3					
Secondary	Posterior Laterals 2 3					
Secondary	Shrugs 1 2 3					

APPENDIX A: WEIGHT-TRAINING PROGRESS CHART						
	DATE →					
	SHOULDERS (cont.)	WT/REPS	WT/REPS	WT/REPS	WT/REPS	WT/REPS
Secondary	External Rotation 1					
	2					
	3					
	BICEPS					
Primary	*Seated Bicep Curls 1					
	2					
	3					
Secondary	Preacher Curls 1					
	2					
	3					
Optional	Reverse Curls 1					
	2					
	3					
	TRICEPS					
Primary	*French Curls 1					
	2					
	3					
Secondary	Tricep Extensions 1					
	2					
	3					
	OR (choose one)					
	Kickbacks 1					
	2					
	FOREARMS					
Primary	Wrist Flexion 1					
	2					
	3					

APPENDIX A: WEIGHT-TRAINING PROGRESS CHART

	DATE →					
	FOREARMS (cont.)	WT/REPS	WT/REPS	WT/REPS	WT/REPS	WT/REPS
Secondary	Wrist Extension 1					
	2					
	3					
Optional	Rope Curl 1					
	2					
	3					
	ABDOMINALS					
Primary	Trunk Curl 1					
	2					
	3					
Optional	Reverse Trunk Curl 1					
	2					
	3					
Optional	Trunk Curl with Rotation 1					
	2					
	3					

USE THIS CHART to monitor the amount of weight you use at each workout. The chart presents a visual outline of the progression in weight for each exercise over a period of time.

For each exercise performed on a given day, mark the weight that is used and the respective number of repetitions for each set next to the 1, 2, and 3 indicated for that exercise. While the weight might increase, the number of reps might stay the same or decrease.

Do not use the weight-training progress chart provided in the book. The progress chart in the book provides the means to monitor your progress over years. It is designed with only enough spaces for about two weeks of data. Therefore, to report your results, you should make copies. You can download a copy of the chart from my website, www.pt2therapy.com.

APPENDIX B: EXERCISE & MUSCLE GUIDE

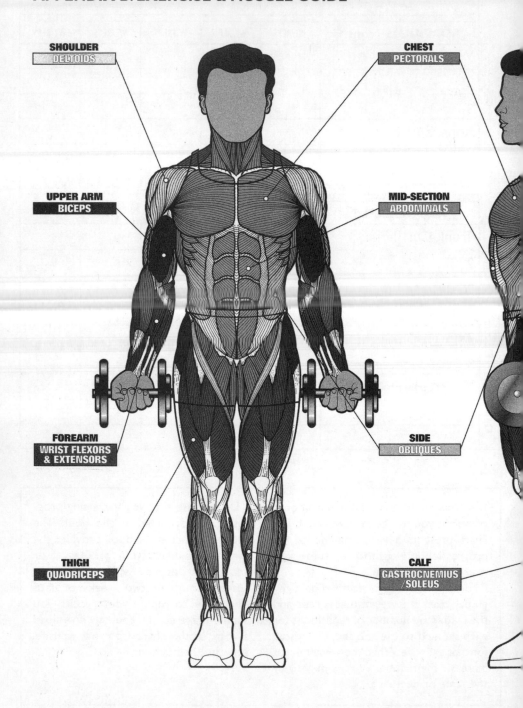

SHOULDER DELTOIDS

CHEST PECTORALS

UPPER ARM BICEPS

MID-SECTION ABDOMINALS

FOREARM WRIST FLEXORS & EXTENSORS

SIDE OBLIQUES

THIGH QUADRICEPS

CALF GASTROCNEMIUS /SOLEUS

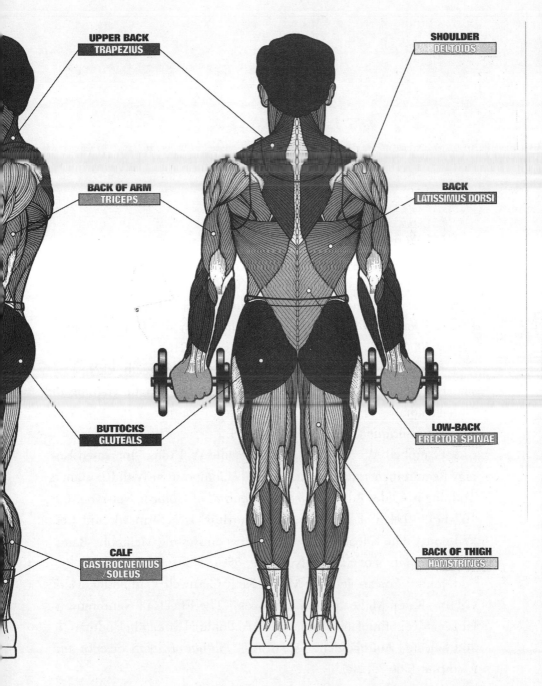

UPPER BACK
TRAPEZIUS

SHOULDER
DELTOIDS

BACK OF ARM
TRICEPS

BACK
LATISSIMUS DORSI

BUTTOCKS
GLUTEALS

LOW-BACK
ERECTOR SPINAE

CALF
GASTROCNEMIUS
/SOLEUS

BACK OF THIGH
HAMSTRINGS

Illustration provided by Algra Corp., www.algra.com.

Notes

1. Judy Foreman, *Globe* staff, "Exercise Appears to Boost Immune System—To a Point," *The Boston Globe*, Health and Science Section, Monday, January 1, 1996, 45. Kevin R. Vincent MD, PhD, Heather K. Vincent, PhD, "Resistance Training for Individuals With Cardiovascular Disease," *Journal of Cardiopulmonary Rehabilitation & Prevention*, July/August 2006, Volume 26 Number 4, Pages 207 216.

2. Fiatarone, M.A.; Marks, E.C.; Ryan, N.D.; Merideth, C.N.; Lipsitz, L.A. and Evan, W.J., 1990. "High-Intensity Strength Training in Nonagenarians, Effects on Skeletal Muscle," *Journal of the American Medical Association*,1990; 263:3029-3034.

3. Campbell, W., M. Crim, V. Young, and W. Evans. "Increased Energy Requirements and Changes in Body Composition With Resistance Training in Older Adults," *American Journal of Clinical Nutrition*, 60: 167-175, 1994. C.E. Broeder, K.A. Burrhus, L.S. Svanevik and J.H. Wilmore, "The Effects of Aerobic Fitness on Resting Metabolic Rate," *American Journal of Clinical Nutrition*, 55: 795-801, 1992.

4. John P. Porcari, Jennifer Miller, Kelly Cornwell, Carl Foster, Mark Gibson, Karen McLean, Tom Kernozek, "The Effects of Neuromuscular Electrical Stimulation Training on Abdominal Strength, Endurance, and Selected Antropometric Measures," *Journal of Sports Science and Medicine* 4: 66-75, 2005.

5. Jun Ding, Anthony S. Wexler, and Stuart A. Binder-Macleod, Interdisciplinary Graduate Program in Biomechanics and Movement Science, Department of Mechanical Engineering, and Department of Physical Therapy, University of Delaware, Newark, Delaware 19716 , 2000. "A Predictive Model of Fatigue in Human Skeletal Muscles," J. Appl. Physiol. 89: 1322-1332.

6. Monica J. Daley and Warwick L. Spinks, Sports Science, Australian Institute of Sport, Canberra, Australian Capital Territory, Australia, Department of Human Movement Studies, University of Technology, Sydney, New South Wales, Australia, "Exercise, Mobility and Aging," *Sports Med* 2000 Jan; 29 (1): 1-12.

7. Maureen C. Jensen, Michael N. Brant-Zawadzki, Nancy Obuchowski, Michael T. Modic, Dennis Malkasian, and Jeffrey S. Ross, "Magnetic Resonance Imaging of the Lumbar Spine in People without Back Pain," the *New England Journal of Medicine* 331:69-73, July 14, 1994.

8. Figure 1 and 2- *Human Physiology: The Mechanisms of Body Function* by Arthur J. Vander, MD, James H. Sherman, PhD, and Dorothy S. Luciano, PhD,Copyright 1990, McGraw-Hill Inc.- Pgs. 290 and 291.

9. Figure 3, 4, 5, 6, 5.5, 5.17, 5.19, 5.35- *Muscle Testing and Function* by Florence Peterson Kendall, PT, and Elizabeth Kendall McCreary, Copyright 1983, Williams & Wilkins, Pgs. 102, 189, 192,193, 209, 92, 94, 99.

About the Author

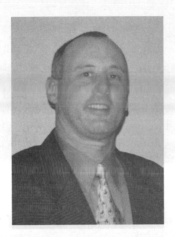

A graduate of the SUNY Health Science Center in Brooklyn, Mitchell Yass is the founder and owner of a thriving physical therapy practice in Farmingdale, NY. Over the past fifteen years, his strength-training program has been used to treat thousands of patients, many of whom were misdiagnosed by x-rays and MRIs. He has served more than 8,000 physical-therapy patients and 4,000 personal training clients at his facility.

Yass was a regular contributor to *Muscle Training Illustrated* and *Fitness Plus* and was named personal trainer of the month by *Exercise for Men Only*. His unique approach and intricate knowledge of human anatomy have been shared through his lectures, the prestigious *Bodies* exhibition in New York, and *Fit for Life!*, the television series he created to help viewers achieve greater levels of fitness throughout life.

A native of Massapequa, Long Island, NY, Mitchell Yass expects to receive his doctorate in physical therapy from the New York Institute of Technology in August 2008. He lives outside New York City

Sentient Publications, LLC publishes books on cultural creativity, experimental education, transformative spirituality, holistic health, new science, ecology, and other topics, approached from an integral viewpoint. Our authors are intensely interested in exploring the nature of life from fresh perspectives, addressing life's great questions, and fostering the full expression of the human potential. Sentient Publications' books arise from the spirit of inquiry and the richness of the inherent dialogue between writer and reader.

Our Culture Tools series is designed to give social catalyzers and cultural entrepreneurs the essential information, technology, and inspiration to forge a sustainable, creative, and compassionate world.

We are very interested in hearing from our readers. To direct suggestions or comments to us, or to be added to our mailing list, please contact:

SENTIENT PUBLICATIONS, LLC
1113 Spruce Street
Boulder, CO 80302
303-443-2188
contact@sentientpublications.com
www.sentientpublications.com